THE RHEUMATOID ARTHRITIS COOKBOOK

AN ANTI-INFLAMMATORY DIET GUIDE AND COOKBOOK WITH OVER 120 EASY RECIPES AND HEALING PLAN FOR INFLAMMATION RELIEF

MONET MANBACCI, PH.D.

(Edition-1)

Copyright © 2020 by Monet Manbacci.

All Right Reserved.

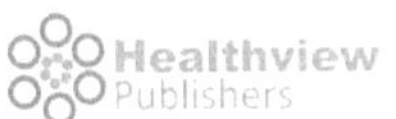

Table of Contents

Inflammation refers to human body's process of fighting against anything that can harm it. This can be a bacterial or virus infections, injuries, or toxins. As the body tries to heal damaged cells due to an attack, human body releases some chemicals that trigger a response from the immune system. This response consists of antibodies and proteins, and increases in blood flow to the damaged cells.

An imbalanced autoimmune response can also create inflammation. In Rheumatoid Arthritis (RA), when an immune system attacks the synovium, which is the lining of the membranes that surround joints, the resulting inflammation can thicken the synovium and destroy the cartilage and bone within the joint. Due to such inflammation, the tendons and ligaments that are responsible for holding joints together will be weakened and stretched. Hence, the joint may lose its shape and alignment by time.

Although it is known that rheumatoid arthritis is a type of an immune disease, other components are involved in creation and triggering the disease. Genetics might be one of the components that may start the RA. Although it is known that genes do not cause RA but that can make human more susceptible to environmental factors such as infections with bacteria or viruses that may be factors of triggering RA. The RA risk factors can be summarized as follows:

- Age: RA can be shown itself at any age but it is most common to start in middle age.
- Sex: women are more vulnerable to develop RA than men.

- Family History: if you have a family member with RA, you are more vulnerable to develop RA compared with a family with no RA patient.
- Smoking: increase the risk of RA development.
- Obesity: overweight people might be at higher risk of developing RA.
- Environment: some exposures to asbestos or silica might increase the risk of RA development.

Some of the first signs of RA include but not limited to:

- Fatigue (lack of energy): this is one of the first signs of RA.
- Slight Fever due to the inflammation
- Weight loss
- Stiffness
- Joint pain
- Joint swelling
- Joint tenderness
- Joint redness

Symmetric pain in multiple joint can occur in people with RA. This is one of the RA signs that makes it different with other joint diseases and other types of arthritis. Although RA symptoms caused by the above-explained factors, research studies have found that many issues can also come from the followings:

- Ignoring signs and symptoms
- Mismanagement of the disorder
- Self-treatment
- Not following the doctor's orders correctly or completely

- Not knowing much about the foods to each and to avoid (a proper diet)
- Not knowing about the impact of anti-inflammatory diet

The last two factors above shows how important a good anti-inflammatory diet can be for people who suffers from rheumatoid arthritis.

One of the best ways to manage your RA, is to follow an anti-inflammatory diet for Rheumatoid Arthritis or a Rheumatoid Arthritis diet, with the help of a comprehensive diet guide and cookbook. This book covers most anti-inflammatory diets such as Medditeranean diet and provides you with the best meal options for RA patients.

This book gives the readers valuable information about healthy nutritional choices, foods to eat or to avoid, food preparation, meal planning, and how to create biweekly cooking plans for people with rheumatoid arthritis. It primarily provide readers with necessary nutritional information and then, guide readers on their cooking and dietary plans. This book is recommended to the groups below:

1. You need to follow the anti-inflammatory diet and want to know how to manage your diet, how to cook varieties of foods, and how to balance your meals using effective meal plans.
2. You have a family member and want to know how to prepare fine meals or make meal plans.
3. You recently realized that you need to follow an anti-inflammatory diet and do not know how to cook for yourself.

4. Your loved one newly diagnosed with rheumatoid arthritis and needs to follow a proper diet.

If you have recently diagnosed or if your loved one have recently diagnosed with rheumatoid arthritis, this book is an excellent source for you to take initial necessary dietary steps, learn how to cook varieties of foods, how to manage your disorder, how to do meal planning and learn about diet tips.

You can imagine how following a bad diet can cause issues when it comes to choosing what you eat and drink. Not only does the condition cause digestive tract irritation and uncomfortable symptoms, but long-term consequences may include malnutrition. To make matters more complicated, your dietary habits may worsen symptoms. Eating and avoiding certain foods explained in this book can help prevent symptom flares. That is why one of the chapters of this book focuses on food preparation and meal planning.

Comprehensive lists of foods to avoid and foods to eat are presented in this book as well. The book then fully covers how to cook for people with rheumatoid arthritis with more than 120 cooking recipes. This chapter covers various types of recipes for breakfast, appetizers, soups, salads, snacks, main courses, desserts, and drinks. Each recipe starts with a brief explanation, preparation time, cooking time, total time, ingredients, instructions, cooking tips, diet-related tips, and nutrition facts. In brief, the chapter provides you with options such as gluten-free, dairy-free, nightshade-free, and bad carbohydrates free recipes that are great for people with rheumatoid arthritis.

The approximated nutrition facts of the recipes in this book have been analyzed by "Verywell fit" Recipe Nutrition

Calculator (Ref: https://www.verywellfit.com). Biweekly cooking plan samples are given in Chapter 6. The same chapter provides you with blank biweekly cooking plan tables for you to write your cooking plans and stick them on your fridge.

It has to be reminded that as each rheumatoid arthritis patient is unique, there is no specific diet or magic diet for everyone. Thus, if you recently diagnosed with RA, the first step for you is to find the best anti-inflammatory diet for yourself and find triggering and non-triggering foods.

Your doctor may provide you with a specific diet related to your inflammation. In this case, you can still use this book as it provides you with lots of anti-inflammatory recipes. You just need to simply avoid foods or ingredients your doctor asks you to avoid and focus more on anti-inflammatory ingredients that are common in the recommended diet by your doctor or nutritionist and the general anti-inflammatory diet explained in this book.

It has to be reminded that the recommendations, hints, and tips provided in this book have been gathered from various related research studies and references from different online/offline resources. These have been found useful by the author of this book, but it does not mean that all will work for you or for your loved one. It should be understood that any recommendations or tips in this book can only be followed only when you take responsibility for it. Be sure that you always talk to your doctor or dietician about the recipes, steps, or hints this book recommends to make sure that they are in line with your health condition.

Chapter 1: Rheumatoid Arthritis Anti-Inflammatory Diet

As explained in the introduction section, there is no specific magic diet for rheumatoid arthritis. However, a modified anti-inflammatory diet with the basis of Mediterranean diet (as presented in this book) might be worthy to try for RA patients. In general, it is recommended for RA patients to follow anti-inflammatory diets.

Your doctors may ask you to combine different diets as well. In this case, you need to follow different diets at the same time. Here, you have to make sure that you consume only foods that are common and safe to consume in diets you follow.

Moreover, many RA patients experience the times that their symptoms are active (or more active). This is called flare-up or flare periods. During this period, more anti-inflammatory ingredients should be added to the diet and all triggering (or even possible triggering) foods should be avoided. Contrariwise, although the inflammation exist a bit, sometimes RA patients feel that their symptoms are gone or the symptoms got better. This is called remission periods. During remission, the RA patients may want to reintroduce some triggering foods to their body again and check their tolerances or consume some debatable foods. In some cases, the RA patients can experience a long remission period and after can experience a relapse or a flare period. Hence, the RA patients need to know the list of foods to consume and to avoid during both remission and flare periods.

The next chapters of this book can help you write your diet plan based on the foods that you can well-tolerated during remission and flare-ups.

In general, the RA patients need to add the following foods in their diet:

- Omega-3 Fatty Acids: this fat can lower the inflammation and cuts down bad LDL cholesterol and triglycerides.
- Beans: are full of fiber that can help lower the C-reactive protein (a sign of inflammation) in your body. They are also great sources of protein, folic acid, magnesium, zinc, and potassium.
- Fruits: some fruits are great for RA patients such as berries, cherries, and dark fruits such as red grapes.
- Nuts: walnuts and soybeans are rich in omega-3 fatty acid.
- Ginger: it has great anti-inflammatory properties.
- Green Tea: is rich in polyphenols, which are antioxidants that can lower the inflammation in your body. Moreover, epigallocatechin-3 can stop production of molecules that lead to the joint damage in RA patients.
- Olive oil: stops the production of chemicals that can cause inflammation.
- Soy: a great source of protein and omega-3 fatty acids.
- Turmeric: an amazing anti-inflammatory spice. The Curcumin that is a compound in turmeric has great anti-inflammatory properties.
- Whole Grains: using whole grains instead of processed one can lower your c-reactive protein. Wholegrains are great source of fiber as well.

- Fresh vegetable such as broccoli and spinach.

In brief, the RA patients need to include omega-3 fatty acids, antioxidants (especially vitamin A, C, E, and selenium), fiber, spices (such as turmeric, ginger, and garlic powder), and flavonoids (berries, green tea, grapes, broccoli, and soy).

On the other hand, the RA patients need to avoid triggering foods. Each patient need to check her/his own tolerance to foods, but in general, the following foods must be avoided:

- Fried and processed foods
- Fast foods
- Lower Advanced Glycation End (AGE) foods: lower the foods that are grilled, fried or pasteurized.
- Sugars and refined carbs
- Aspartame
- Dairy products
- Alcohol and tobacco
- Salt
- Preservatives and flavor enhancers
- Corn oil
- Significantly reduce red meats
- Lower Omega-6 fatty acids
- Gluten: some (not all) experts believe that people with RA should avoid gluten in their diet.
- MSG (Monosodium Glutamate): can trigger the inflammation in body. Avoid salty Asian foods or sauces such as soy sauce, salty snacks and crackers.

CHAPTER 2. COMPREHENSIVE LIST OF FOODS TO EAT AND TO AVOID

This chapter provides comprehensive lists of foods to eat and foods to avoid for patients who wants to follow anti inflammation diet for rheumatoid arthritis. Different food categories are investigated, and the tips related to flare-up and remission periods are explained.

As explained before, each patient is unique and there is no unique magic diet for all patients with rheumatoid arthritis. Hence, you always need to consult with your doctor and check if recommended anti-inflammatory foods explained in this chapter is fine for you or not. Also, always test your tolerance regarding foods, have your research and, if you decide to consume, have them in in moderation at the beginning to test your tolerance better.

FRUITS

In general, fruits with anti-inflammatory properties are avocado, strawberries, blueberries, raspberries, grapes, blackberries, cherries, pomegranate, watermelon, and orange. Other great fruits to consume are banana, cantaloupe, honeydew melon, and papaya. Always check your tolerances with your doctor before consuming these fruits.

During Flares

1. In many cases, poached, skin and core-removed fruits can be well-tolerated.

2. Make sure you do not consume poached fruits, or compotes high in sugar during flares.
3. Do not forget to add explained anti-inflammatory fruits in your diet.
4. Check if a fruit increases symptoms during flare-up periods or not. If yes, avoid eating it.
5. Check if the fruit is easy to digest or not. If it is hard to digest, avoid eating it during flares.
6. Check if the fruit can help dehydration or not. Consider other factors when you choose a fruit to eat during flares.
7. If you are fructose-intolerant, use only fruits without fructose.
8. In general, black-colored fruits such as black grapes, blackberries, and blueberries are recommended for rheumatoid arthritis patients.
9. Some patients may find citrus fruits triggering as it has high acidity, which may triggers inflammations.

During Remissions

1. You can consume fruits during flare-ups, but it is recommended to peel off and remove cores of fruits during the remission period as well.
2. Most fruits can be well-tolerated during remission periods.

VEGETABLES

In general, green leafy vegetables, such as spinach, kale, broccoli, and Brussel sprouts are great anti-inflammatory vegetables. However, some patients with chronic inflammation cannot consume leafy greens. Other great vegetables to consume are carrot, cucumber, ginger root, zucchini, butter lettuce, and beets. If you can consume such vegetables, these are great for healing inflammations. Tomato is another great anti-inflammatory vegetable. However, many patients with rheumatoid arthritis should not use tomatoes as it is triggering. Other nightshades such as eggplant, zucchini, and potato might also not be tolerated by some rheumatoid arthritis patients. Always check your tolerances with your doctor before consuming these vegetables.

During Flares

1. In many cases, boiled or steamed, skin-removed vegetables can be well-tolerated.
2. Make sure you do not stir fry vegetables.
3. Eat vegetables in moderation during flares.
4. Check if a vegetable increases symptoms. If yes, avoid eating it.
5. Check if a vegetable has anti-inflammatory properties or not. Consider other factors when you chose a vegetable to eat during flares.
6. Consuming purple (or red) potato or sweet potato is recommended instead of using russet potatoes.
7. Garlic and onion are good for rheumatoid arthritis patients. However, check your tolerance before consuming them.

During Remissions

1. It is recommended to consume tolerable vegetables (raw or boiled) during the remission period.
2. Many vegetables can be well-tolerated during remission periods.
3. Remember to eat vegetables in moderation.

4. Try to consume vegetables with fiber, folic acid, vitamin A, C, E, and K, calcium, and other required nutrients.

HERBS AND SPICES

In general, here are the great herbs for rheumatoid arthritis diet:

- Turmeric (Curcumin)
- Ginger
- Cinnamon
- Peppermint
- Cayenne
- Black Pepper
- Chili Pepper
- Mint
- Garlic powder
- Onion powder
- Lemonzest
- Rosemary
- Cloves
- Green Tea
- Ginseng
- Cat's claw
- Willow Bark
- Frankincense
- Chili Peppers
- Resveratrol
- Angelica
- Saffron
- Cardamom

Some patients with rheumatoid arthritis may find some of the above herbs triggering (especially chili peppers or cayenne). Always check your tolerances with your doctor or nutritionist before consuming herbs and spices.

During Flares

1. Remember to eat herbs and spices in moderation during flares.
2. It is fine to boil or steam herbs and consume during flares.
3. Check if an herb or spice has anti-inflammatory properties or not. Consider other factors when you chose an herb to consume during flares.
4. Avoid consuming salt. If your doctor allows you to consume salt in moderation, try to consume Himalayan Salt.

During Remissions

1. Many herbs and spices can be well-tolerated during remission periods.
2. Use more herbs and spices with anti-inflammatory properties and rich in nutrients and vitamins during remission periods.

OILS

Here are the recommend lists of oils for RA inflammation:

- Extra virgin olive oil
- Avocado oil

Other nut-based oils such as walnut oil and grapeseed oil might be used in moderation.

It is recommended to consume organic high quality, and less refined types of extra virgin olive oil.

During Flares

1. It is highly recommended to avoid consuming lots of oil during flare-up periods. Most meals should be boiled or cooked without consuming oils.
2. A safe option for cooking during flares is using extra virgin olive oil in moderation.
3. Avocado and fish oils are also other safe options. Make sure that the oil you consume does not contain high amounts of Omega-6.

During Remissions

1. It is recommended to avoid consuming palm and corn oils.
2. Always try to consume high-quality organic oils.
3. Remember that the best options are extra virgin olive oil and avocado oil.
4. Check your tolerance if you want to cook your meal with any other types of oils.

ANIMAL PROTEINS

In general, low-fat, skin-removed lean/extra lean cuts should be used. It is recommended to avoid or significantly reduce the amount of red meat taken each month and use other sources of proteins. It is highly recommended to consume ostrich meat instead of beef/lamb meat.

During Flares

1. Avoid eating skins and fat cuts.

2. Avoid eating cold cuts.

3. Avoid eating spicy cold cuts.

4. Avoid eating hard to digest meats.

5. Avoid eating animal proteins with the skin.

6. Eat animal proteins in moderation.

7. Use lean or extra lean cuts for red meat and pork if you can tolerate them during flares.

8. The ostrich is an excellent source of protein to try during flares.

9. Grass-fed meats are recommended as they have higher sources of proteins and vitamins compared with grain-fed meats.

10. Poaching and boiling eggs are the best methods of making eggs during flare-up periods. Do not consume fried eggs.

During Remissions

1. Remove skins of poultries and other animal proteins before consumption.

2. Stick to lean and extra lean cuts during remission periods as well.

3. Remember to eat animal proteins in moderation.

4. Try to limit red meats in your meal plan.

5. Put high amounts of proteins from poultry in your weekly meal plan.

6. Avoid consuming fatty parts of meat, chicken, and pork during remission periods, as well.

SEAFOOD

1. Seafood is an excellent source of healthy fatty acids for RA patients. It contains Omega-3 that may help reduce joint pain and swelling.

2. Remember to consume seafood in moderation during flare-up periods.
3. It is recommended to put fish at least twice a week in your diet.

Some of the greatest seafoods to eat include but not limited to: Tune, Salmon, Trout, Halibut, Sardines, Herring, Mackerel, Shrimps, and prawns.

WHOLE GRAINS

In general, wholegrains are safe for patients with rheumatoid arthritis.

1. Oatmeal can be a great source of insoluble fiber for RA patients.
2. Oatmeal family and quinoa can be consumed if they can be tolerated well.
3. Always consult with your doctor if you can consume gluten products or not. If you are gluten intolerant or cannot eat gluten, stick to none-gluten products.

REFINED GRAINS

In general, refined carbohydrates such as white bread and pastries should be avoided in RA diet.

1. White rice should be avoided.
2. It is not recommended to consume grain products with corn.
3. It is recommended to consume non-refined organic, and non-GMO grains.

GLUTEN-FREE FLOUR OPTIONS

1. Many gluten-free flours might not be tolerated well. It is recommended to avoid consuming gluten if it is possible.
2. On the contrary, many gluten-free flour options can be well-tolerated.
3. Flours from nuts should be well-grounded.
4. Almond flour, walnut flour, amaranth flour, tapioca and cassava flour are some of recommended gluten-free flours.

NUTS

Nuts such as almonds and walnuts are great for healing RA inflammation. However, it is very important to talk to your doctor before consuming any nuts. You need to make sure that putting nuts in your diet is safe for you. For instance, people with other health conditions such as IBD cannot not use nuts at all.

1. Some nuts such as almond can be used in moderation in other forms such as smoothened almond butter or almond milk (if they can be well-tolerated).
2. Make sure the almond butter or other nut butter you want to consume is smooth.
3. You can also make stews with well-ground nuts such as walnut if you can tolerate them.

SEEDS

Seeds such as pumpkin seeds are great for healing inflammation. However, it is very important to talk to your doctor before consuming any seeds. You need to make sure that putting seeds in your diet is safe for your health condition.

LEGUMES

Legumes can be used in general. However, some patients with other specific disorders should avoid consuming legumes. Consume fully cooked legumes only if you can tolerate and if they are matched with your health conditions.

1. Check your tolerance level when you want to consume legumes shown in yellow color.
2. It is recommended to consume organic legumes.

SWEETENERS

1. It is highly recommended to avoid consuming artificial sweeteners.
2. All refined sugars such as white sugar should be avoided.
3. Patients need to check their tolerance for natural plant-based sweeteners such as, stevia, honey, maple syrup or agave syrup.
4. It seems that Stevia can be well-tolerated. However, use it in moderation during flare-up periods.
5. Avoid consuming aspartame as well.

DAIRY PRODUCTS

1. It is highly recommended to avoid consuming dairy products.
1. Some RA patients without lactose intolerance are able to consume milk, goat milk, kefir, yogurt and yogurt drinks during remission periods in moderation. This group of patients needs to avoid consuming fatty dairy products such as cheese even during remission. It is also recommended for this

group of patients to put yogurt and kefir in their meal plan as they are excellent sources of probiotics and prebiotics, respectively.

2. Lactose-intolerant patients need to avoid consuming dairy products such as yogurt with lactose, even during remission periods. Alternatively, they can eat lactose-free plain yogurts.

BUTTER

1. It is highly recommended to avoid consuming butter during flare-up periods.
1. Patients in remission may consume butter in limited amounts. However, it is recommended to consult with your doctor and check your tolerance when consuming it.
2. It is also recommended not to consume salted butter.
3. The best-recommended butter option for those who allowed to use or can tolerate butter during remission periods is organic grass-fed unsalted butter.

CHEESES

It is highly recommended to avoid consuming cheese products during flare-up and remission periods.

SAUCES, DIPS, AND GRAVIES

During Flares

1. Avoid eating greasy and fatty sauces/gravies.
2. Avoid eating spicy sauces/gravies.
3. Avoid consuming high sugar gravies/sauces.

4. Avoid eating sauces or gravies with triggering ingredients.
5. Avoid ketchup and Mayo.
6. Avoid eating hard to digest sauces/gravies.
7. Remember to eat ready gravies/sauces in moderation.
8. Avoid consuming sauces/gravies with dairy inside during flares.

During Remissions

1. Eat gravies/sauces in moderation.
2. Always make healthy and fresh gravies/sauces.
3. It is recommended to consume low-fat, low-sodium organic mayo sauces.
4. Avoid ketchup.
5. Avoid spicy sauces/gravies even during remission periods.

READY FOODS (IN GENERAL)

During Flares

1. Avoid eating greasy and fatty foods (e.g., fast foods).
2. Avoid eating foods with triggering ingredients.
3. Avoid eating hard to digest foods.
4. Avoid eating foods with refined sugar.
5. Avoid eating processed and canned foods.
6. Avoid processed meats such as hotdogs or sausages
7. Remember to eat ready foods in moderation.
8. Avoid consuming fried foods (especially deep-fried) such as chips, and fries.

9.   Avoid consuming BBQ and grilled foods.

During Remissions

1.   Always try to consume fresh and healthy foods.
2.   Foods with healthy fats are also suitable for patients with RA.
3.   Foods rich in soluble fiber and high in protein are excellent choices during remission periods.
4.   Avoid eating triggering foods, even during remission periods.

OTHER FOODS TO EAT OR TO AVOID

- Dark chocolate is a great anti-inflammatory option. However, you should consult with your doctor and check your tolerance before consumption.
- Some patients with RA found nightshades such as tomatoes, potatoes, and eggplants problematic. It is recommended to avoid consuming nightshades during flares.
- Mushroom is great for anti-inflammatory diet, however, some patients found it triggering. Always check your tolerance before consuming mushrooms.
- Remember that added sugars as well as salts are not recommended for people with RA.
- Energy drinks and drinks with high amounts of sugars (both with white sugar and with artificial sweeteners) should be avoided.

CHAPTER 3. RHEUMATOID ARTHRITIS COOKING TECHNIQUES AND DIET

Each patient with rheumatoid arthritis is unique in terms of symptoms, complications, and food intolerances. That is why there is not a single magic diet for everyone and that is why each person need to find her/his triggering foods and avoid consuming them. However, there are great foods and vegetables with anti-inflammatory properties that should be added to your diet to reduce inflammation and help relieve rheumatoid arthritis symptoms.

COOKING STYLES/METHODS

1. The best cooking methods for patients who wants to follow the anti-inflammatory diet are boiling, steaming, roasting, poaching, stewing, and air frying.
2. It is crucial not to fry (especially deep fry) foods during flare-up periods. If you want to fry, simmer or cook on a pan, spray a bit of extra virgin olive oil or avocado oil. Even you can spray it when roasting.
3. When cooking beef or poultry, make sure the inside of your meat cooked well. Always try to cook well-done.
4. You can poach fruits and boil vegetables and other meals to consume. These are the best cooking methods during flares. If you are poaching fruits, make sure you are not using any sources of refined sugar. If you need a substitute for sugar, you can try stevia. Other possible

options are honey, maple syrup, and agave syrup. Remember to consume such alternatives only if you can tolerate them well.

5. Air frying is one of the best options for you if you want to have skin-removed purple potato chips or zucchini chips. Consume a small amount of extra virgin olive oil when you want to air fry by an air fryer.

6. Broiling is another method that is might be fine with some patients during remissions. However, patients should avoid eating the burned parts of broiled foods.

7. In brief, the best cooking methods for patients with rheumatoid arthritis during flares/relapses are boiling/poaching and steaming. During remission, other cooking methods such as roasting and stir frying might be used with cautious by consuming a truly little amount of oil. The recommended oil to use is an extra virgin olive oil and avocado oil (if available, buy high-quality organic types).

FOOD INGREDIENTS

FRUITS AND VEGETABLES

Fruits and vegetables contain valuable sources of nutrients that are essential. When you have rheumatoid arthritis, you have to make sure that you eat fruits and vegetables that are very easy to digest and can sooth your inflammation.

1. Try to add the best fruits and vegetables for rheumatoid arthritis explained in the previous

chapter to your diet. Making a fruit salad is a great meal option for you.

2. During a severe flare-up, it is recommended to consume skin-removed poached/boiled fruits instead of raw fruits.

3. During a severe flare-up, boil or steam vegetables that are easier to digest, such as broccoli, or asparagus.

4. Try to avoid consuming fruit and vegetable seeds a lot.

5. Try to avoid juices with added sugars.

6. One of the greatest options for juicing fruits and vegetables is to use a sturdy juicer or a juicing machine especially if you need to take a low fiber diet due to your health condition. When you are juicing with such devices, you are removing the fibers of fruits and vegetables but you absorb vitamins, minerals, and other healthy properties of fruits and vegetables. This method is fabulous for patients who should follow a low-fiber diet.

7. The best fruit and vegetable juices for many patients are berries, grapes, cantaloupe, melon, papaya, pomegranate, lemon, broccoli, and spinach.

RICE, NOODLE AND PASTA

1. If you can tolerate fiber, you may want to try brown rice. Avoid using white rice.

2. To make an excellent rice meal, steamed brown rice in a rice cooker or a proper pot. It is recommended to add a teaspoon of turmeric powder to the boiling water to have a beautiful anti-inflammatory yellowish rice!

3. Alternatively, you can make zucchini noodles or spiralized zucchini using a spiralizer if you can tolerate zucchini.
4. Whole wheat pasta is a great meal option for rheumatoid arthritis patients who can tolerate gluten is it contains selenium.
5. Cook your pasta according to its package instruction. Typically, you need to choose a proper pot and pour water on top of your pasta to cover all pasta. After boiling water, cook pasta in the boiling water for about 10 minutes. You can add extra virgin olive oil to the boiling water to taste. Use them in moderation. As mentioned before, try to avoid white pasta.
6. Adding some fresh ginger into the boiling water of pasta is recommended.
7. You can consume gluten-free pasta options with brown rice flour or quinoa.
8. Alternatively, you can make spaghetti squash to have a delicious healthy vegetarian spaghetti.

MEAT AND POULTRY

Animal proteins contain various types of vitamins, proteins and minerals, such as vitamin-B, E, zinc, magnesium, and iron. They also have amino acids that are essential for people with rheumatoid arthritis. That is why they need to consume proteins from different sources. In general, red meat is not recommended for rheumatoid arthritis patients.

1. Do not use processed meats at all. Consuming meats that have been salted, fermented, smoked, or canned is not recommended. Avoid consuming cold-cuts and sausage products.

2. Significantly reduce the amount of red meat you eat every week.

3. You can have extra lean or lean red meat in moderation. Choose low-fat or no-fat cuts.

4. During flares, avoid red meat intake.

5. Do not stir fry meat and poultry. Cook them well in boiling water.

6. Avoid consuming fatty parts of any kind of meat.

7. Ostrich meat without fat might be one of the best red meat options for you. The ostrich meat has a similar taste of beef meat, but with lower fat and cholesterol. Moreover, it is rich in protein, iron, and calcium that might worthy to try.

8. Do not eat spicy or fatty meat products such as salami and pepperoni especially during flares.

9. You can cook chicken/turkey breasts, legs, and thighs. Make sure the skins are removed. It is not recommended to eat chicken wings during flares.

10. Use low-fat (or no fat) extra lean (or lean) part of pork.

11. Avoid eating bacon during flares. Significantly reduce consuming it during remission periods as well.

SEAFOOD

Seafood is another excellent source of protein, amino acids, and healthy fats. Oily fish such as salmon, mackerel, trout, and sardines contain healthful fats, including omega-3 fatty acids. This combat inflammation and may help reduce the risk of heart disease and certain cancers. Health experts often recommend eating at least two servings of oily fish per week. These can include trout, salmon, mackerel, herring, tuna, and sardines.

1. To keep fat levels as low as possible, bake them with small amounts of extra virgin olive oil. It is the best way to cook the fish, for easy digestion.
2. Tuna is another excellent seafood that patient may want to consume. You can make a delicious sandwich with tuna, avocado, and lemon juice. It is not recommended to eat raw sashimi such as tuna sashimi, especially if you are not sure about the place you purchased them, as you will be more vulnerable to diseases such as salmonella.
3. Well-cooked shrimps, prawns, and crabs can also be consumed.

GRAINS

Grains are excellent sources of fiber, vitamin-B, iron, and other healthy nutrients such as magnesium and selenium. In general, grains contain three components: germ, bran, and endosperm. Whole grains have all three components, but refined grains have a process of removing the germ and bran to have a smooth texture. During this process, some iron and B-vitamin can be removed from the grain. As such, some recommend consuming whole grain products during remission if you can tolerate and if you are entirely sure that you do not have any other complications such irritable bowel syndrome (IBS).

1. Avoid consuming refined grains such as white bread, pasta or rice, corn flour, all-purpose flour, waffles, rice snacks and cream of wheat. Instead use whole wheat breads, brown rice, and oatmeals.
2. Almond flour is an excellent option for cooking and baking especially for those who are gluten intolerant.
3. Ready-to-eat cereals especially instant oatmeals might be a good option.

4. Remember that gluten-intolerant patients need to avoid gluten and alternatively consume non-triggering non-refined gluten-free products.

Soy, Eggs, and Tofu

1. Soy, eggs, and tofu are great sources of protein. Also, egg yolks contain high amounts of vitamin D, and people with rheumatoid arthritis are often deficient in vitamin D and A.
2. In addition to lean protein, soy and tofu contain bioactive peptides, and some research suggests that these have antioxidant and anti-inflammatory properties, which may help manage your disease.
3. Do not eat fried eggs or scrambled eggs during flares. Hard-boil eggs is a method for eating eggs.
4. When you are in a flare, bake firm tofu instead of stir-frying it.

Dairy Products

1. Many yogurts contain probiotics, which are healthy bacteria that may help reduce inflammation in the gut. Kefir is also another great option with anti-inflammatory, antioxidant, and anti-microbial properties. You may want to put yogurts and kefir in your diet only if you can tolerate lactose.
2. Although dairy products are rich in calcium, and manufacturers may fortify them with vitamins D and C, many however, contain lactose, a type of sugar, and some doctors recommend eliminating lactose from the anti-inflammatory diet as it can be hardly digested. Milk may irritate the tissue around the joints as well. Hence, it is recommended to avoid consuming dairy product. A study in 2017 showed

milk anti-inflammatory effects in patients that can tolerate cow milk. As the result of this study conflicts with other expert's recommendation, consult with your doctor if you want to drink milk. One recommendation is to eliminate cow milk for couple of weeks and then, reintroduce it to check your body response to it.

3. The number of dairy servings per day may depend upon the individual dietary needs of a person. As explained, many people with rheumatoid arthritis found dairy products worsen their symptoms. If not the case, a person may try 1 serving or less of the following options at the beginning of the reintroduction stage:
    - Cheese (goat cheese can be a good option)
    - Lactose-free Milk
    - Yogurt with live active cultures

4. Lactose-intolerant patients should avoid any forms of lactose in their meals. It is also recommended for patients that are not lactose intolerant to limit consuming lactose. Suggested alternatives are:
    - Almond milk
    - Oat milk
    - Soy milk

SPICES AND HERBS

1- Certain spices can be used in your cooking. Turmeric, ginger, and cinnamon are fantastic spices for meals as they have anti-inflammation and anti-microbial properties.

2- Salt should be avoided. If you want to consume salt, you need to consult with your doctor and ask if consuming salt is safe for your health condition.

3- Black pepper can be used in general.

4- Other hot spicy peppers such as cayenne or red pepper are fine in general, but check your tolerance before consuming them.

5- Garlic and onion powders are fine in general. However, check our tolerance before consumption.

6- It is recommended to grate ginger instead of mincing it.

7- Other recommended herbs that can be used in moderation are: frankincense, willow bark, and saffron

8- Lemon zest can be used during remission in moderation.

9- Some studies show anti-inflammatory properties of ginseng, as well. You may want to use it in moderation if you can tolerate it well.

10- Use other common herbs such as basil, cilantro, rosemary, Angelica, and parsley in moderation if you can tolerate.

CHEESE

1- Avoid high-fat daily products such as cheese.

2- It is recommended to limit your low-fat cheese intake.

3- Some patients may tolerate goat cheeses. You can check if you can tolerate goat cheese or not.

Remember that it is recommended to avoid consuming cheese or consume small amounts of low-fat lactose-free cheese products during remission periods.

OILS

1- The best oil recommended is extra virgin olive oil.

2- Avoid consuming butter during flare-ups.

3- Avocado oil is another recommended oil to use for cooking.

4- Safflower oil, grapeseed oil, sunflower oil, vegetable oil, and soybean oil are excellent sources of Omega-6, which is great for the proper inflammatory response. However, patients with rheumatoid arthritis need to avoid consuming Omega-6 a lot.

SAUCE, GRAVY, SALAD DRESSINGS

Here are some of the essential tips for using sauce, gravy, and salad dressings:

- Do not use hot spicy sauces, gravies, or salad dressings.

- Mayonnaise might be used in moderation in remissions only. Try to make or purchase low-fat low-sodium organic types.

- Avoid ketchup.

- Many of patients cannot tolerate tomato-based products such as tomato sauce, and tomato paste. Check your tolerance level for these types of sauces before consuming them. It is recommended to avoid using them.

- Mustard: should be fine in general. Use in moderation if you are unsure that you can tolerate it well.

- Sour cream: avoid sour cream in general. Instead, you may want to use probiotic yogurt.

- Smooth low-fat low-sodium sauces and salad dressings are fine in general. Always try to check your tolerance first, and if you are okay, use them in moderation.

- Gravies: low-sodium low-fat gravies from poultry is generally fine to consume in moderation.
- Soy sauce is not recommended as it contains Mono-sodium glutamate (MSG), which can trigger inflammation.
- Balsamic vinegar: try to check your tolerance first, and if you are okay, only use it in moderation.
- White vinegar: try to check your tolerance first, and if you are okay, only use it in moderation.
- Apple cider vinegar: some believe it can help reduce inflammation. No scientific evidences have been found. You may want to check our tolerance first and consume apple cider vinegar in moderation.
- Red/White wines: avoid using wine in sauces or dressings.
- Tahini: is fine in general. Always try to check your tolerance first, and if you are okay, use it in moderation.
- Barbecue (BBQ) sauce: has a high acidity level. Check your tolerance first, and if you are okay, use it in moderation.
- Garlic and onion gravies: organic low sodium types are recommended.
- Honey and maple syrup are fine in general. Always try to check your tolerance first, and if you are okay, use them in moderation.

DRINKS

Drink options are fully explained as a chapter section in this book. In general, patients should avoid sodas and fizzy beverages. As coffee is debatable, you may want to avoid drink it during flare-ups and limit having it during remissions. Some herbal teas such as peppermint and green tea are great alternatives for caffeinated beverages. Alkaline water is another great drink you can have. You can simply squeeze a fresh lemon to your drinking water.

MEALS

BREAKFAST

Breakfast is an essential meal for everyone. Typically, the breakfast of people with rheumatoid arthritis should be rich in proteins and soluble fibers. Soluble fibers are easier to digest as they can absorb water and become like gels during the digestion process. Some prefer to consume foods with more carbohydrates in the morning, and some who are more concern about their weight gain want to consume foods with fewer carbohydrates for their breakfast. If you're going to have more carbs, you can consume sweet fruits that you can tolerate. Some of the great breakfast options are:

- Decaffeinated hot drinks (coffee, tea, etc.)
- Eggs: Boiled eggs are recommended.
- Oatmeal: you can combine oatmeal with cinnamon, honey (If you can tolerate), applesauce, cherries or skin-removed cubed apples to have a very delicious oatmeal breakfast.
- Banana oatmeal
- Almond butter (smoothened) sandwich
- Avocado sandwich
- Unsweetened yogurts with berries
- Preferably use lactose-free yogurt with skin-removed raw or poached fruits such as berries, papaya, pear, peach, and banana.

SOUPS

Soup is one of the great meals you can add in your diet. Perfectly blended soups are very easy to digest and are great for patients who should have a liquid diet or Bland diet, and for patients with specific chronic inflammatory conditions. Soups can be added more in your meal plan during flare-up periods. Some of the most exceptional soups for people who wants to follow RA diet are:

- Blended or mashed zucchini soup (if you can tolerate nightshades)
- Pumpkin soup
- Butternut squash soup
- Chicken noodle soup

SALADS

Salad is a great meal for people with rheumatoid arthritis. You can mix different types of ingredients with different high nutrients, vitamins, and minerals together in a salad. However, making a salad could be challenging, as many typical salad ingredients are not good for some RA patients with chronic inflammation. This book provides you with many delicious salad recipes in Chapter-5. Some fantastic salad options and salad ingredients for people with rheumatoid arthritis include but not limited to:

- Skin-removed cucumber and carrot.
- Fruit salad can be made from certain fruits recommended for patients with rheumatoid arthritis.
- Zucchini, purple potato, whole wheat pasta, and chicken are other great ingredients for having a delicious salad.

- Other salad ingredients such as spinach, broccoli, parsley, and basil can be used if you can tolerate them.
- Some patients cannot tolerate vegetables that contain histamine, such as spinach. Always check your tolerance, as your doctor about triggering foods and adjust your diet them.

SNACKS

Snacks can play a crucial role in the meal plan of patients with rheumatoid arthritis as it is recommended for them to eat smaller meal portions five or six times during a day. Hence, a full, healthy snack that cannot trigger the inflammation can be beneficial. Here are some of the snack options (if you can tolerate):

- Hummus
- Applesauce
- Avocado sandwich
- Non-refined Gluten-free snacks
- Fruits (poached or compote)
- Oatmeal
- Quinoa bar
- Zucchini chips (if you can tolerate)
- Almond milk
- Dark chocolate (only if you can tolerate)

DESSERTS

Dessert can also be an excellent meal for patients with rheumatoid arthritis. Here are some of the dessert options:

- Ice creams (sorbets) made only with recommended fruits and not with cow milk.

- Shakes made with recommended fruits and almond or soy milk
- Trifle with banana and lemon
- Gluten-free cakes
- Applesauce
- Fruit compote or bowl made with recommended fruits and not with refined sugars.

SIDE DISHES

Each meal can have its well-matched side dishes. Some of the side dish options include, but not limited to:

- Boiled purple potatoes or sweet potatoes in moderation
- Boiled leafy vegetables such as spinach (if you can tolerate). Broccoli, kale, Brussel sprouts are great vegetable options.
- Zucchini as chips (skin removed and if you can tolerate)
- Cooked, raw or glazed carrots
- Mushroom: Check your tolerance first and then consume in moderation if you are fine. If not, you may use shiitake mushroom alternatively.
- Beets: are great side dishes in general. Check your tolerance before consumption.
- Green beans are fine. Check your intolerance first and use it in moderation if you can tolerate it.
- Avocado: mashed or cubed is an excellent side dish for you.
- Lemon or lime wedges
- Recommendation: try not to use tomatoes, caramelized onion, roasted garlic, and corn.
- Sauerkraut is another good option for you.

- Pickles: you may want to consume pickles in moderation only if you can tolerate them well.

CHAPTER 4. FOOD PREPARATION & MEAL PLANNING

The following tips can help you have an effective food preparation and meal planning for your rheumatoid arthritis:

EATING HABITS

1- Eat smaller portions, but frequent meals 5 to 6 times a day.
2- Keep yourself hydrated. Drink plenty of water and other allowed juices during a day. Pump-up your electrolyte intake, especially during flares using low-sugar sports drinks or make yours at home.
3- Drink slowly and chew well.
4- Do not use straw as you may ingest air, which can lead to produce gas.
5- You can drink recommended herbal teas after your meal for better digestion, especially if you think that you ate a heavy meal.
6- Give time to your herbal tea to brew well.
7- Eat your meal in peace and comfort in a relaxed place. Do not talk too much when you are eating your meal.
8- Do not work with your phone or laptop while eating your meals.
9- Do not drink water when you are eating meals.
10- Do not skip your breakfast at all.
11- Do not starve yourself. Assign specific times for your meals and stick to those times.
12- Do not eat very late. Eat dinner at least 2 hours before your sleep time, or 4 hours after your lunch.

13- Always have a meal plan and follow it. The worst thing for you is not knowing what to eat and what to cook.

14- Reduce consuming alcohol, sugar, and coffee. Avoid consuming them in flare-up periods.

15- Do not leave your foods at normal temperature for more than 2 hours.

16- Avoid deep-fried, unhealthy, fatty, and greasy foods.

GROCERY SHOPPING

1- To prepare your meals in advance, you need to create a list before you go out for daily or weekly shopping.

2- The list should include ingredients you need for your daily or weekly cooking plan. Remember that the ingredients you purchase should be well-tolerated.

3- Always try to purchase organic, non-GMO products.

4- Always try to buy lower-fat/no fat products.

5- For eggs, try to purchase organic and free-range type

6- For meat or pork, stick to grass-fed low-fat lean (or extra lean) cuts.

7- Use ostrich meat as an alternative to other red meats.

8- For poultry, low fat (or fat-free) skin-removed breasts and legs are the best options.

9- For cheese, try to purchase low-fat lactose-free options. Use cheese in moderation.

10- For milk and yogurts, always purchase unsweetened and unflavored types of plant-based milks such as almond milk or soy milk. Use milk in moderation. Avoid drinking cow milk.

11- For grains, try to find gluten-free options. Stick to gluten-free options.

12- For bread, try to find gluten-free bread that is not highly processed.

13- For baking, purchase gluten-free flours such as almond flour.

14- Purchase fruits and vegetables that you can tolerate well.

15- For oil, purchase extra virgin olive oil. Avocado oil is another great option.

16- Keep having turmeric, ginger and cinnamon in your kitchen cabinet.

17- Avoid purchasing processed foods.

18- For sauces such as mayonnaise, try to purchase organic low fat and low sodium types. Use mayo in great moderation. Avoid ketchup.

19- Always purchase organic potatoes. Stick to red/purple potato.

20- It is not recommended to purchase fruit juices with added sugar, and juices from concentrate. The best option for you is to make a juice from non-triggering fruits at home.

21- If you want to purchase almond butter, get the organic and smooth one.

22- To make your meals sweet, avoid any types of refined sugar. You may want to try stevia.

23- If you can tolerate honey, try to consume organic, raw, and non-pasteurized honey. Consume non-pasteurized honey with cautious and always consult with your doctor first.

24- Maple syrup in limited amount (1 tbsp) may work for you as a sweetener option.

25- Purchase fresh foods instead of frozen or canned foods.

26- Read the ingredients of the snacks you may want to purchase. Make sure you can tolerate all ingredients well.

27- It is very important to avoid consuming products with High Fructose Corn Syrup (HFCS).

COOKING TOOLS

You do not need to buy any specific tools to follow a diet for rheumatoid arthritis, but here are some tools that can help you ease the cooking process:

1- <u>Cast Iron skillet:</u> some people suggest having an iron skillet to absorb iron better.
2- <u>Blender:</u> for those who can use nuts in moderation, they need to blend them well. Having a suitable blender/mixer can help you cook well-blended meals such as soups, smoothies, nut butter, and juices.
3- <u>Juicer:</u> having a powerful juicer can help you taking the juices of fruits and vegetables. With this tool, you may have fruits or vegetables that you cannot tolerate due to their high insoluble fiber.
4- <u>Small lunch-dinner boxes:</u> it is recommended to eat smaller portions six times a day. One great idea to follow this eating style is to provide lunch, snacks, and dinners in separate boxes. For instance, you can put your lunch in two small lunch boxes instead of a big one, and eat each box in different time (e.g., with two hours of time-difference) at your workplace.
5- <u>Spiralizer:</u> to have spaghetti-like zucchini, potatoes, and pumpkin, you may want to use a spiralizer.
6- <u>Air fryer:</u> air frying can be a great cooking option, as it does not need to consume much oil. You can make great zucchini or potato chip snacks or other meals using an air fryer.
7- <u>Timer and thermometer:</u> both are helpful tools for you to cook delicious meals. Remember that meats

should be cooked well, and these tools can help you checking this.

KITCHEN PREPARATION

Here are some of the tips to prepare yourself and your kitchen before cooking:

1. Wash your hands perfectly when you want to cook.
2. Always wash fruits and vegetables before using them.
3. Remember not to consume fruit cores or vegetable seeds a lot. Wash skin fruits carefully.
4. Wash meats before cooking. Use disposable gloves when washing meats and put gloves in the garbage after. Always wash your hands with warm water right after washing meats and poultries.
5. Use a separate cutting board for raw meat.
6. Keep raw meats away from other foods in the kitchen and fridge.
7. Never mix cooked foods with raw meats. Mixing can happen in plates, cutting boards, etc. Never eat such foods.
8. Remember to cook or boil meats, seafood, and vegetables in perfection.
9. Keep the kitchen area (especially countertop) well-cleaned and sanitized.

MEAL PLANNING

1- Use proper cooking methods explained in this book. Keep your cooking style simple:
    a. If you are in remission (it seems that your symptoms are gone for couple of months (although exist)), you are free to apply

cooking techniques such as stir-fry foods by spraying a bit of extra virgin olive oil.

    b.   If you are in a flare, try to stick to techniques such as boiling, steaming, and poaching.

    c.   Consuming freshly grated spices such as ginger and turmeric is better than consuming their powders.

2- You should have your meal plans ready. Use the information on this book to create your meal plans. The plans should include only foods that you can tolerate.

3- You also should know the strategy of finding triggering foods for yourself. To keep it simple, if you eat a specific food for a short period and observed any symptoms such as joint pain, swollen joint, joint stiffness, fatigue, fever, and joint tenderness you might be intolerant to that particular food. If you ate a meal and you are not sure about the ingredient(s), you have to write this meal in your journal and record your symptoms and conditions there. Next, you need to review your journal at the end of each week or two again and check if you can find any relations or common ingredient between different meals that you could not tolerate. You can visit a dietitian or a nutritionist to guide you more on how to find triggering foods. Different rheumatoid arthritis patients have different triggering foods to avoid. The most debating foods include but not limited to nightshades such as tomato, eggplant, zucchini and potato, coffee, and white rice.

4- Create at least two, bi-weekly meal plans, with adequate variety and stick to them according to your health condition.

The next chapter of this book gives excellent cooking recipes for rheumatoid arthritis patients.

Chapter 5. Cooking Recipes for Rheumatoid Arthritis Patients

This chapter provides you with more than 120 fantastic delicious cooking recipes for people with rheumatoid arthritis. It consists of various recipes to cook, serve, and enjoy, such as breakfasts, soups, salads, appetizers, main courses for lunch and dinner, desserts, drinks, and snacks.

Each cooking recipe starts with a brief introduction, preparation time, cooking time, total time, serving size, ingredients, instructions, cooking tips, Diet-related Tips, and nutrition facts. It has to be noted that the approximate nutrition facts of the recipes in this book have been analyzed by "Verywell fit" Recipe Nutrition Calculator.

Breakfasts

Gluten-Free Fluffy Pancake

A great gluten-free pancake for those who cannot tolerate gluten.

- Prep Time: 5 minutes
- Cook Time: 10 minutes
- Total Time: 15 minutes
- Serving: 4

Ingredients:

- 2 organic, free-range eggs
- 2 cups almond flour
- 2 cups kefir
- 1 teaspoon lime juice

- 1.5 tablespoon baking powder

<u>Instructions</u>

1. In a medium bowl, mix and whisk all ingredients.
2. Heat a large pan with extra virgin olive oil and cook both sides of pancakes until golden over medium heat.
3. Enjoy!

<u>Cooking Tips:</u>

- You can use maple syrup or honey with your pancakes if you can tolerate it.

Nutrition Facts

Servings: 4

Amount per serving

Calories	402
	% Daily Value*
Total Fat 7.3g	9%
Saturated Fat 3.5g	17%
Cholesterol 97mg	32%
Sodium 132mg	6%
Total Carbohydrate 71.2g	26%
Dietary Fiber 3.4g	12%
Total Sugars 6.3g	
Protein 11.5g	
Vitamin D 8mcg	39%
Calcium 20mg	2%
Iron 1mg	4%
Potassium 93mg	2%

Banana and Apple Pancakes

Another yummy lactose-free, gluten-free pancake for those on rheumatoid arthritis anti-inflammatory diet.

- Prep Time: 5 minutes
- Cook Time: 10 minutes
- Total Time: 15 minutes
- Serving: 2

<u>Ingredients</u>

- 1 apple, skin-removed
- 3 bananas, cubed
- 4 medium-sized organic, free-range eggs
- 2 cups almond flour
- 1 tablespoon extra virgin olive oil
- Honey or maple syrup (optional)

<u>Instructions</u>

1. In a medium bowl, mash and whisk apple, bananas, and eggs.
2. Heat a large pan with high-quality extra virgin olive oil, flatten your pancake and cook both sides until golden over medium heat.
3. Serve with honey if you can tolerate it. Enjoy!

<u>Cooking Tips:</u>

- You can use maple syrup or honey with your pancakes if you can tolerate it.

Nutrition Facts

Servings: 2

Amount per serving

Calories	**401**
	% Daily Value*
Total Fat 16.5g	21%
Saturated Fat 3.9g	20%
Cholesterol 327mg	109%
Sodium 126mg	5%
Total Carbohydrate 56.5g	21%
Dietary Fiber 7.3g	26%
Total Sugars 33.9g	
Protein 13.3g	
Vitamin D 31mcg	154%
Calcium 56mg	4%
Iron 3mg	14%
Potassium 871mg	19%

Eggs, Salmon, and Avocado

This breakfast contains a great source of healthy fats and protein. A smooth, fast, and delicious breakfast recipe to cook!

- Prep Time: 5 minutes
- Cook Time: 10 minutes
- Total Time: 15 minutes
- Serving: 2

Ingredients:

- 2 scrambled or boiled eggs
- 2 oz salmon, cooked or canned
- 1 avocado
- 1 teaspoon extra virgin olive oil

Instructions

1. Heat a large pan with high-quality extra virgin olive oil, and scramble your eggs over medium heat.
2. Mix your scramble with avocado cubes and small salmon pieces. Enjoy!

Cooking Tips:

- You can also mash your avocado instead of cubing it.

Diet-related Tips:

- If you are in a flare, do not scramble eggs. Instead, use boiled salmon and eggs.

Nutrition Facts

Servings: 2

Amount per serving

Calories   **353**

	% Daily Value*
Total Fat 30.4g	39%
Saturated Fat 6.7g	34%
Cholesterol 182mg	61%
Sodium 107mg	5%
Total Carbohydrate 9.6g	3%
Dietary Fiber 6.7g	24%
Total Sugars 1.4g	
Protein 13.5g	
Vitamin D 44mcg	220%
Calcium 26mg	2%
Iron 2mg	9%
Potassium 677mg	14%

BAKED APPLE

For those who have RA, cooked, and raw fruits are great breakfast ingredients. You can use this recipe for cooking fruits like apple, peach, and pear.

- Prep Time: 5 minutes
- Cook Time: 40 minutes
- Total Time: 45 minutes
- Serving: 2

Ingredients

- 1 teaspoon cinnamon
- 1 teaspoon extra virgin olive oil
- 2 cups of water
- 1 tsp stevia
- 2 apples, cored

Instructions

1. In a medium/large pot, boil your apple with cinnamon, olive oil, water, and stevia over high heat for 40 minutes.
2. Remove the apple skin, and then, enjoy!

<u>Cooking Tips:</u>

- You can use the same instruction to make baked fruits such as pear or peach.

<u>Diet-related Tips:</u>

- Remember: Do not use white sugar. Simply use stevia (one tablespoon).

Nutrition Facts

Servings: 2

Amount per serving

Calories	173

	% Daily Value*
Total Fat 2.7g	4%
Saturated Fat 0.3g	2%
Cholesterol 0mg	0%
Sodium 12mg	1%
Total Carbohydrate 40.6g	15%
Dietary Fiber 6g	21%
Total Sugars 32g	
Protein 0.7g	
Vitamin D 0mcg	0%
Calcium 27mg	2%
Iron 1mg	6%
Potassium 256mg	5%

Pear Oatmeal Bars

A great source of fiber for those who have RA. This bar is gluten and lactose-free with a great taste of pear and ginger.

- Prep Time: 10 minutes
- Cook Time: 25 minutes
- Total Time: 35 minutes
- Serving: 4

<u>Ingredients</u>

- 4 organic pears
- ½ cup applesauce
- 1 teaspoon ground ginger

- ½ teaspoon salt (only if you are allowed and you can tolerate)
- ½ cup organic smooth almond butter
- 2 teaspoons pure vanilla extract
- 2 teaspoons ground cinnamon
- ¾ teaspoon baking powder
- ¾ cup oat or quinoa flour (or gluten-free flour)
- ½ cup rolled oats (or a small package of ready oatmeal)

Instructions

1. Preheat oven to 375 °F.
2. Cook the pear or use a pear compote. Blend your pears to make a puree.
3. Mix your pear puree with applesauce, salt, almond butter, ginger, vanilla extract, cinnamon, baking powder, flour, and oats.
4. Pour your mix into a suitable oven pan.
5. Bake your oatmeal for 25 minutes until inside cooks well. Cut the baked oatmeal like bars.
6. Let it be cooled first and then serve!

Cooking Tips:

- It is recommended to use organic oats or ready oatmeal.
- To check if the inside cooks well, insert a toothpick inside. If it comes out without sticking to your bar, it shows that it cooked well.

Diet-related Tips:

- Cook your pear or use pear compote if you cannot tolerate raw pear.

Avocado & Egg Breakfast Toast

A very simple, delicious breakfast dish, high in protein and healthy fat.

- Prep Time: 5 minutes
- Cook Time: 10 minutes
- Total Time: 15 minutes
- Serving: 2

<u>Ingredients</u>

- 4 slices of toast or gluten-free bread
- 1 avocado
- 2 large organic free-range eggs
- 4 egg whites
- 1 tablespoon lime juice
- Pepper to taste

<u>Instructions</u>

1. Toast your bread the way you want.
2. Mix eggs, egg whites, and pepper in a bowl and scramble it in a pan over medium heat for 7 minutes.

3. Coat your toasts with scrambled mix and mashed avocado. Then, squeeze lime. Enjoy!

Diet-related Tips:

- Boil your eggs if you are experiencing a severe flare-up.
- You can add a bit of low-fat feta cheese if you can tolerate during remission periods.

Nutrition Facts

Servings: 2

Amount per serving

Calories	411
	% Daily Value*
Total Fat 26.4g	34%
Saturated Fat 6.5g	32%
Cholesterol 191mg	64%
Sodium 467mg	20%
Total Carbohydrate 21.2g	8%
Dietary Fiber 7.2g	26%
Total Sugars 2.5g	
Protein 24.7g	
Vitamin D 18mcg	88%
Calcium 103mg	8%
Iron 2mg	12%
Potassium 751mg	16%

SMOOTHIE BOWL

A mix of skin-removed and chopped fruits can create a tremendous rich breakfast!

- Prep Time: 10 minutes
- Cook Time: 0 minutes
- Total Time: 10 minutes
- Serving: 2

Ingredients

- 1 banana, sliced
- 1 cup almond milk
- 1 cup papaya chunks

- 1 cup diced mango

<u>Instructions</u>

1. Blend all mentioned ingredients in a blender. Serve and Enjoy!

<u>Cooking Tips:</u>

- You can use the same instruction to make fruit bowls with other fruits you can tolerate.
- You can add 1 cup of papaya to your bowl as well.

Nutrition Facts

Servings: 2

Amount per serving

Calories	419
	% Daily Value*
Total Fat 29.2g	37%
Saturated Fat 25.5g	128%
Cholesterol 0mg	0%
Sodium 20mg	1%
Total Carbohydrate 43.3g	16%
Dietary Fiber 6.6g	24%
Total Sugars 30.6g	
Protein 4.5g	
Vitamin D 0mcg	0%
Calcium 42mg	3%
Iron 2mg	14%
Potassium 755mg	16%

ZUCCHINI BREAD OATMEAL

Enjoy the taste of grated zucchini and oatmeal and have a healthy breakfast!

- Prep Time: 5 minutes
- Cook Time: 7 minutes
- Total Time: 12 minutes
- Serving: 2

<u>Ingredients</u>

- ⅓ cup organic rolled oats or ready oatmeal

- 1 cup unsweetened almond milk
- ½ teaspoon cinnamon powder
- ½ cup zucchini
- 1 teaspoon vanilla extract
- Maple syrup (optional)

Instructions

1. Mix your milk with cinnamon and oat in a medium pot and boil the mixture over medium heat for 4 minutes.
2. Grate zucchini, add it to the mix, and stir well for three minutes.
3. In a small bowl, mix vanilla extract and maple syrup.
4. When oatmeal cooked, remove from heat and pour the syrup on it.
5. Let it be cooled and then serve!

Cooking Tips:

- You can use maple or agave syrup in this recipe if you can tolerate.

Nutrition Facts

Servings: 2

Amount per serving

Calories — **82**

% Daily Value*

Total Fat 2.7g	3%
Saturated Fat 0.3g	2%
Cholesterol 0mg	0%
Sodium 94mg	4%
Total Carbohydrate 11.5g	4%
Dietary Fiber 2.2g	8%
Total Sugars 0.9g	
Protein 2.6g	
Vitamin D 1mcg	3%
Calcium 162mg	12%
Iron 1mg	6%
Potassium 222mg	5%

BREAKFAST FRUIT SALAD

A mix of a variety of fruits (skin-removed and chopped) can create an excellent breakfast salad for people with rheumatoid arthritis!

- Prep Time: 5 minutes
- Cook Time: 25 minutes
- Total Time: 30 minutes
- Serving: 6

Ingredients

- 2 large firm bananas, cubed
- 1 medium mango, skin removed and cubed
- 1 medium green apple, skin removed and cubed
- 1 medium papaya, skin-removed and cubed
- 1 tablespoon lemon juice
- 1 tablespoon stevia (optional)
- ⅓ cup orange juice (optional)

Instructions

1. Mix all fruits in a bowl.
2. Boil your orange juice, lemon juice, and stevia in a small pot (over high heat). Stir well.
3. Let the juice be cooled. Then, add your cooled juice to the fruit bowl. Enjoy!

Cooking Tips:

- You can use orange juice in this recipe if you can tolerate it.

Diet-related Tips:

- If you are experiencing a severe flare-up, you can remove the skin and cook your fruits.

Nutrition Facts

Servings: 6

Amount per serving		
Calories		**108**
		% Daily Value*
Total Fat 0.4g		1%
Saturated Fat 0.1g		1%
Cholesterol 0mg		0%
Sodium 6mg		0%
Total Carbohydrate 27.7g		10%
Dietary Fiber 3.5g		13%
Total Sugars 18.8g		
Protein 1g		
Vitamin D 0mcg		0%
Calcium 17mg		1%
Iron 1mg		3%
Potassium 331mg		7%

BANANA SPLIT OATMEAL

A great combination of oatmeal and banana can make a great breakfast full of fiber and potassium.

- Prep Time: 10 minutes
- Cook Time: 0 minutes
- Total Time: 10 minutes
- Serving: 2

Ingredients

- ½ cup water, almond milk
- 1 cup old-fashioned rolled oats or a small ready oatmeal package
- ½ banana, cubed

Instructions

1. Boil your milk or water in a pot over high heat.
2. Add oat to it. Stir for two more minutes.
3. Serve your oatmeal with cubed bananas. Enjoy!

<u>Cooking Tips:</u>

- You can use honey, maple or agave syrup in this recipe if you can tolerate.

Nutrition Facts

Servings: 2

Amount per serving

Calories	**319**

	% Daily Value*
Total Fat 17.1g	22%
Saturated Fat 13.2g	66%
Cholesterol 0mg	0%
Sodium 89mg	4%
Total Carbohydrate 37.8g	14%
Dietary Fiber 6.2g	22%
Total Sugars 6g	
Protein 7.1g	
Vitamin D 0mcg	0% ·
Calcium 32mg	2%
Iron 3mg	16%
Potassium 412mg	9%

EGG TACOS WITH AVOCADO

Enjoy a breakfast sandwich with egg and avocado, which is full of healthy fats and functional proteins.

- Prep Time: 5 minutes
- Cook Time: 10 minutes
- Total Time: 15 minutes
- Serving: 2

<u>Ingredients</u>

- 4 small tortillas
- 2 organic, free-range eggs
- 1 avocado

<u>Instructions</u>

1. Warm or toast tortillas.
2. Boil your eggs.
3. Mash your avocado

4. Fill your tortillas with avocado and eggs. Enjoy!

<u>Diet-related Tips:</u>

- If you are sensitive to gluten, use soft gluten-free bread instead of tortillas.

Nutrition Facts

Servings: 2

Amount per serving

Calories	373
	% Daily Value*
Total Fat 25.3g	32%
Saturated Fat 5.7g	29%
Cholesterol 164mg	55%
Sodium 167mg	7%
Total Carbohydrate 30.4g	11%
Dietary Fiber 9.8g	35%
Total Sugars 1.3g	
Protein 10.2g	
Vitamin D 15mcg	77%
Calcium 74mg	6%
Iron 2mg	11%
Potassium 636mg	14%

CRISPY HASH BROWN WITH EGG

Start your day with hash brown and egg! A great combination, as always!

- Prep Time: 20 minutes
- Cook Time: 15 minutes
- Total Time: 35 minutes
- Serving: 2

<u>Ingredients</u>

- 2 large red or purple potatoes, shredded
- ¼ cup gluten-free flour such as almond flower
- 2 tablespoons extra virgin olive oil
- 2 organic range-free eggs
- Pepper to taste

<u>Instructions</u>

1. Shred potatoes and rinse them until the water cleared. Dry potatoes.
2. Mix your potatoes with flour, eggs, and pepper.
3. Flatten your mix in a large skillet and let it cook over medium heat until golden brown. Flip and cook the other side.
4. Remove from the skillet and drain with a paper towel. Enjoy!

Cooking Tips:

- To flip it quickly, you can cut in half or quarter.

Diet-related Tips:

- Try to boil and mash your potatoes well during flares and use this recipe only if you can tolerate purple or red potato.

Nutrition Facts

Servings: 2

Amount per serving

Calories	385
	% Daily Value*
Total Fat 18.7g	24%
Saturated Fat 3.4g	17%
Cholesterol 164mg	55%
Sodium 70mg	3%
Total Carbohydrate 45.9g	17%
Dietary Fiber 2.8g	10%
Total Sugars 3g	
Protein 10.2g	
Vitamin D 15mcg	77%
Calcium 34mg	3%
Iron 2mg	12%
Potassium 686mg	15%

GRILLED ALMOND BUTTER HONEY BANANA SANDWICH

An excellent easy to make a sandwich for your breakfast.

- Prep Time: 5 minutes
- Cook Time: 0 minutes

- Total Time: 5 minutes
- Serving: 2

Ingredients

- 1 tablespoon extra virgin olive oil
- Few grams of almond butter
- 1 banana
- 4 slices of wholegrain bread (if you can tolerate) or gluten-free bread
- Honey or maple syrup to taste

Instructions

- Toast your bread slices, as you desired.
- Mash banana, coat your bread with banana, almond butter, and honey (maple syrup). Enjoy!

Cooking Tips:

- You can use honey, maple or agave syrup in this recipe if you can tolerate.

Diet-related Tips:

- Make sure you are using smoothened types of almond butter.

Apple Cinnamon Oatmeal

Enjoy tasting a traditional apple cinnamon oatmeal that can be prepared in less than 15 minutes.

- Prep Time: 5 minutes
- Cook Time: 15 minutes
- Total Time: 20 minutes
- Serving: 2

Ingredients

- 1 tablespoon extra virgin olive oil
- 1 cup gluten-free ground oats or ready oatmeal
- 2 cups unsweetened almond
- ½ teaspoon cinnamon
- 1 large apple, sliced and skin-removed
- 1 tablespoon maple syrup, or agave syrup
- ¼ cup pomegranate juice (optional)

Instructions

- Preheat oven to 375 °F.

- In a medium bowl, mix and whisk oats with cinnamon, oil, apple, pomegranate juice (optional), maple syrup, and milk.
- Use a suitable baking pan or sheet. Spread your mix to it and bake for 15 minutes until golden brown.

<u>Cooking Tips:</u>

- You can prepare this breakfast in a large skillet over medium heat for 10-15 minutes until brown.
- Use agave syrup or 1 teaspoon of stevia if you cannot tolerate maple syrup or honey.

<u>Diet-related Tips:</u>

- Use pomegranate juice only if you can tolerate it.

Nutrition Facts

Servings: 2

Amount per serving

Calories	276
	% Daily Value*
Total Fat 12.5g	16%
Saturated Fat 1.3g	7%
Cholesterol 0mg	0%
Sodium 182mg	8%
Total Carbohydrate 40.6g	15%
Dietary Fiber 6.5g	23%
Total Sugars 17.6g	
Protein 4.8g	
Vitamin D 1mcg	7%
Calcium 323mg	25%
Iron 3mg	15%
Potassium 332mg	7%

APPETIZERS

TURKEY POTPIE SOUP

Great soup with perfect ingredients for people with rheumatoid arthritis.

- Prep Time: 10 minutes

- Cook Time: 35 minutes
- Total Time: 45 minutes
- Serving: 4

Ingredients

- ¼ cup gluten-free flour (e.g., almond flour)
- 16 oz turkey breast, cubed
- 2 cups turkey/chicken stock, divided
- 4 cups almond milk
- 1 teaspoon turmeric powder
- 2 celery stalks, chopped in small pieces
- 1 large carrot, cubed 1 inch (~2.54 cm)
- 2 medium purple or red potatoes, peeled and cubed 1 inch (~2.54 cm)
- Pepper, to taste

Instructions

1. Mix 1 cup of turkey/chicken broth with flour and whisk well. Set aside.
2. Pour another cup of broth into a large pot. Add turkey, celery, potatoes and turmeric powder inside and boil until vegetables and turkey get soft.
3. Warm milk and add to the mix. Then, add carrots and cook for another 5 minutes. Add Pepper to taste.

Cooking Tips:

- You may want to add one cup of mushroom if you can tolerate it.
- You can remove flour from the recipe if you do not have one or do not want a soup with a thick texture.

- You can make this soup with chicken breasts as well.

<u>Diet-related Tips:</u>

- If you cannot tolerate ordinary mushrooms, you may try Shiitake mushroom.
- If you cannot tolerate potatoes, simply remove it from the recipe.

Nutrition Facts

Servings: 4

Amount per serving	
Calories	**326**

	% Daily Value*
Total Fat 2.4g	3%
Saturated Fat 0.5g	3%
Cholesterol 54mg	18%
Sodium 1696mg	74%
Total Carbohydrate 42.3g	15%
Dietary Fiber 4.2g	15%
Total Sugars 18.6g	
Protein 30.6g	
Vitamin D 1mcg	6%
Calcium 341mg	26%
Iron 3mg	16%
Potassium 1286mg	27%

Potato-Ginger Miso Soup

A fabulous Miso soup with great healing properties. A great source of required vitamins and minerals for people with rheumatoid arthritis:

- Prep Time: 10 minutes
- Cook Time: 30 minutes
- Total Time: 40 minutes
- Serving: 3-4

<u>Ingredients</u>

- 1 fresh ginger or ½ tablespoon fresh grated ginger
- 2 cups sodium-free/low sodium vegetable broth

- 2 tablespoons miso
- 2 medium red or purple potatoes, peeled and cubed 1 inch (~2.54 cm)
- ½ cup unsweetened almond milk

<u>Instructions</u>

1. Boil potatoes in a medium pot until softened.
2. Drain and mash your potatoes.
3. In a medium/large pot, mix broth, and ginger, and boil over medium heat.
4. Add mashed potatoes to the mix and blend until smoothened.
5. Add warm miso and almond milk. Blend again until smoothened. Then, heat the soup for 5 more minutes over medium heat. Enjoy!

<u>Cooking Tips:</u>

- You can add 1 cup of chicken breast to the recipe if you want to have chicken miso.

<u>Diet-related Tips:</u>

- Do not use this recipe if you cannot tolerate potatoes.

Nutrition Facts

Servings: 3

Amount per serving	
Calories	**242**

	% Daily Value*
Total Fat 11.3g	15%
Saturated Fat 8.9g	45%
Cholesterol 0mg	0%
Sodium 951mg	41%
Total Carbohydrate 28.8g	10%
Dietary Fiber 5g	18%
Total Sugars 4.2g	
Protein 8g	
Vitamin D 0mcg	0%
Calcium 33mg	3%
Iron 2mg	12%
Potassium 857mg	18%

PARSNIP/CARROT SOUP

The parsnip is a root vegetable from the carrot family. Instead of parsnip, you can use carrot in the recipe.

- Prep Time: 10 minutes
- Cook Time: 30 minutes
- Total Time: 40 minutes
- Serving: 4

<u>Ingredients</u>

- 1 celery stalk, chopped
- 4 parsnips or carrots, cubed 1 inch (~2.54 cm)
- 3 cups chicken broth
- 1 tablespoon extra virgin olive oil
- 2 red or purple potatoes, skin removed and cubed 1 inch (~2.54 cm)
- 1 teaspoon pepper

<u>Instructions</u>

6. Choose a large pan and cook celery and parsnip (carrot) using extra virgin olive oil over medium heat and occasionally mix until semi-soft texture.

7. Warm up the broth and pour it into the pan. Add potato, and pepper (optional) and cook for 20 minutes.
8. Enjoy the soup as it is or blend it for having a puree.

<u>Cooking Tips:</u>

- You can mix all ingredients at the same time and let it boil for 25-30 minutes.

<u>Diet-related Tips:</u>

- Do not use parsnip if you cannot tolerate it, or you are experiencing a severe flare-up. Instead, use carrots.
- If you cannot tolerate potatoes, simply remove it from the recipe.

Nutrition Facts

Servings: 4

Amount per serving

Calories	**184**

% Daily Value*

Total Fat 4.9g	6%
Saturated Fat 0.9g	4%
Cholesterol 0mg	0%
Sodium 593mg	26%
Total Carbohydrate 29.7g	11%
Dietary Fiber 6g	21%
Total Sugars 5.1g	
Protein 6.3g	
Vitamin D 0mcg	0%
Calcium 45mg	3%
Iron 1mg	7%
Potassium 864mg	18%

PUMPKIN SOUP

Great semi-classical pumpkin soup can be one of your choices to make every week.

- Prep Time: 15 minutes
- Cook Time: 15 minutes

- Total Time: 30 minutes
- Serving: 4-6

Ingredients

- 2 lbs (~1 kg) pumpkin, skin-removed, seeds-removed, chopped
- 1 large carrot, skin-removed, diced
- 2 medium red or purple potatoes, skin removed, diced
- 4 cups sodium-free/low sodium chicken broth
- ½ cup soy milk or almond milk
- Pepper, to taste

Instructions

1. Mix and boil all ingredients in a large pot over medium heat.
2. Remove from heat. Blend the soup until smooth.
3. Add pepper to taste

Cooking Tips:

- You can cook vegetables first in a large skillet by 1 tablespoon extra virgin olive oil over medium heat until semi-soft texture. Then, boil and blend.

Nutrition Facts

Servings: 6

Amount per serving

Calories 174

% Daily Value*

Total Fat 1.5g	2%
Saturated Fat 0.5g	3%
Cholesterol 0mg	0%
Sodium 543mg	24%
Total Carbohydrate 34.3g	12%
Dietary Fiber 7.6g	27%
Total Sugars 8.5g	
Protein 7.8g	
Vitamin D 0mcg	1%
Calcium 86mg	7%
Iron 3mg	17%
Potassium 988mg	21%

Diet-related Tips:

- If you cannot tolerate potatoes, simply remove it from the recipe.

STRACCIATELLA SOUP

This delicious Italian soup is entirely in line with patient tolerance levels full of healthy ingredients. It can significantly supply your protein.

- Prep Time: 10 minutes
- Cook Time: 15 minutes
- Total Time: 25 minutes
- Serving: 4

Ingredients

- 6 cups low sodium/sodium-free chicken broth
- 2 tablespoons semolina flour or gluten-free flour
- 3 large organic free-range eggs
- Pepper, to taste
- 1 tablespoon fresh parsley (optional)

Instructions

1. In a large pot and over high heat, bring chicken stock to simmer. Add Pepper.
2. In a large bowl, whisk eggs, and semolina or gluten-free flour altogether.
3. Slowly pour the egg mixture into your pot and simmer well. Let the soup simmer.
4. Serve and garnish it with parsley if you want. Enjoy!

Nutrition Facts

Servings: 4

Amount per serving

Calories	164

	% Daily Value*
Total Fat 8.3g	11%
Saturated Fat 3.5g	18%
Cholesterol 147mg	49%
Sodium 1277mg	56%
Total Carbohydrate 5.5g	2%
Dietary Fiber 0.2g	1%
Total Sugars 1.3g	
Protein 15.4g	
Vitamin D 13mcg	66%
Calcium 120mg	9%
Iron 2mg	9%
Potassium 376mg	8%

HAM AND CELERY SOUP

A delicious soup for people with rheumatoid arthritis who love ham.

- Prep Time: 10 minutes
- Cook Time: 20 minutes
- Total Time: 30 minutes
- Serving: 4

<u>Ingredients</u>

- 2 large red or purple potatoes, peeled and cubed 1 inch (~2.54 cm)
- 1 cup cooked ham, diced and cubed 1 inch (~2.54 cm)

- 3 cups sodium-free/low sodium chicken broth
- 1 tablespoon extra virgin olive oil
- ¼ cup gluten-free flour
- ½ cup celery stalk, diced
- 2 cups almond milk
- Pepper to taste

<u>Instructions</u>

1. Boil potatoes, celery, ham, and chicken broth in a large pot over medium heat for 15 minutes.
2. In a large pan, pour high-quality extra virgin olive oil and whisk flour over medium heat. Stir consistently until golden brown. Warm milk and add slowly to the flour. Stir continuously for five minutes.
3. Pour the mix into the pot and stir. Add Pepper to taste. Enjoy!

<u>Cooking Tips:</u>

- For having a classic taste, you can use honey ham.

<u>Diet-related Tips:</u>

- If you are in a severe flare-up, avoid using ham/honey ham. Instead, use fat-removed pork tenderloin or chicken breasts.
- Use red potatoes only if you can tolerate it. If not, simply remove it from the recipe.

Nutrition Facts

Servings: 4

Amount per serving

Calories 316

% Daily Value*

Total Fat 9.2g	12%
Saturated Fat 3.1g	15%
Cholesterol 29mg	10%
Sodium 935mg	41%
Total Carbohydrate 43.3g	16%
Dietary Fiber 5.3g	19%
Total Sugars 8.2g	
Protein 16.1g	
Vitamin D 1mcg	3%
Calcium 190mg	15%
Iron 2mg	12%
Potassium 1112mg	24%

BUTTERNUT SQUASH SOUP

A perfect soup for people with rheumatoid arthritis to be included in their weekly diet.

- Prep Time: 10 minutes
- Cook Time: 55 minutes
- Total Time: 65 minutes
- Serving: 6

Ingredients

- 3 lbs (~1.5 kg) butternut squash, halved & skin-removed
- 2 carrots, peeled and cubed
- 3-4 cups low sodium chicken or vegetable stock/broth
- ¼ cup olive oil (for roasting option)
- 1 teaspoon ground black pepper, to taste (optional)

Instructions

1. Boil all ingredients in a large pot over medium heat for 40 minutes until softened. Remove from the pot. Allow to cool down for 5-10 minutes.

2. Pour all ingredients into a blender. Then, blend until smooth. Serve hot and enjoy!

<u>Cooking Tips:</u>

- Be careful with the steam that may come out of the blended soup.

Nutrition Facts
Servings: 6

Amount per serving

Calories   **193**

% Daily Value*

Total Fat 8.7g	11%
Saturated Fat 1.3g	7%
Cholesterol 0mg	0%
Sodium 1037mg	45%
Total Carbohydrate 29.3g	11%
Dietary Fiber 5g	18%
Total Sugars 6.2g	
Protein 3.6g	
Vitamin D 0mcg	0%
Calcium 117mg	9%
Iron 2mg	10%
Potassium 869mg	18%

Chicken Noodle Soup

The chicken noodle soup is one of the famed soups all around the world. Enjoy making it in less than 45 minutes!

- Prep Time: 5 minutes
- Cook Time: 40 minutes
- Total Time: 45 minutes
- Serving: 6

<u>Ingredients</u>

- 1 cup vermicelli or egg noodles (gluten-free option)
- 8 skin-removed chicken legs
- 2 cups of water
- 1 tablespoon extra virgin olive oil
- 2 large carrots, cubed & skin-removed

- 1 celery stalk, chopped
- 6 cups low sodium chicken stock/broth
- 1 teaspoon ground black pepper, to taste (optional)
- ¼ cup fresh parsley, chopped (optional)

Instructions

1. In a large skillet, heat high-quality olive oil over medium heat and cook celery and carrots for 5 minutes.
2. Pour chicken broth into the skillet, add and cook chicken legs.
3. Add crushed bouillons and water to cover all ingredients.
4. When chicken cooked, use a plate to shred it and remove the bone.
5. Bring shredded chickens back to the soup and add noodles. Add pepper. Cover it for 7 minutes. Then, open the lid and stir well.
6. Serve in a bowl and garnish with chopped fresh parsley (optional)

Cooking Tips:

- You can use skin-removed chicken thighs or breasts instead of chicken legs, as well.
- You have to use gluten-free noodles if you are gluten-intolerant.

CREAMY CHICKEN SOUP

A very delicious savory soup specially modified for people with rheumatoid arthritis.

- Prep Time: 5 minutes
- Cook Time: 30 minutes
- Total Time: 35 minutes
- Serving: 4-6

<u>Ingredients</u>

- 1.5 lbs boneless, skin-removed chicken breast
- 1 cup carrots, skin-removed and cubed 1 inch (~2.54 cm)
- 1 medium red or purple potato, skin-removed and cubed 1 inch (~2.54 cm)
- 2 tablespoons extra virgin olive oil
- 1 cup almond milk
- 3 cups low-sodium chicken broth
- 1 teaspoon turmeric powder
- Pepper, to taste
- ½ teaspoon dried thyme
- 1-2 tablespoon(s) lemon juice

- 1 cup mushrooms (optional)

Instructions

1. Heat extra virgin olive oil in a large pot and cook chicken over medium heat with turmeric, and pepper until golden brown both sides. Remove chickens.
2. Add carrots, potato, thyme, and mushroom (optional) to the pot. Stir well until half-cooked. Add chicken broth. Then, let it cook for 15-20 minutes.
3. Add warm milk and 1-2 tablespoon(s) lemon juice. Let it simmer for five more minutes. Serve warm and enjoy!

Cooking Tips:

- You can use ½ cup shiitake mushroom if regular mushrooms irritate your gut, or remove mushroom from the recipe.

Diet-related Tips:

- If you are in extreme flare-up, boil chicken as well.
- Use red potatoes only if you can tolerate it. If not, simply remove it from the recipe.

Nutrition Facts

Servings: 6

Amount per serving

Calories	**224**
	% Daily Value*
Total Fat 6.7g	9%
Saturated Fat 1g	5%
Cholesterol 68mg	23%
Sodium 145mg	6%
Total Carbohydrate 10.9g	4%
Dietary Fiber 1.4g	5%
Total Sugars 3.4g	
Protein 29.6g	
Vitamin D 21mcg	106%
Calcium 61mg	5%
Iron 2mg	8%
Potassium 285mg	6%

SEAFOOD CHOWDER SOUP

A must-try recipe if you are in love with seafood!

- Prep Time: 10 minutes
- Cook Time: 25 minutes
- Total Time: 35 minutes
- Serving: 4-6

Ingredients

- 2 medium red or purple potatoes, peeled and cubed 1 inch (~2.54 cm)
- 2 cups of low-sodium vegetable broth or chicken broth
- ¾ cup of soy milk
- 4 oz salmon filet, peeled and cubed
- 4 oz codfish filet, peeled and cubed
- 8 raw shrimps, peeled
- 2 tablespoons fresh lemon juice
- 1 bay leaf
- ½ teaspoon grated ginger
- Pepper to taste

Instructions

1. In a large pot, warm chicken broth and add potatoes, bay leaf, salmon, and cod.
2. Let the soup cook for 15 minutes over medium heat. Stir occasionally. Cover but leave a corner open for the steam to escape.
3. Add warm milk, shrimp, lemon juice, ginger, and pepper to the soup. Stir for 5-10 minutes. Enjoy!

Cooking Tips:

- You can add ⅓ cup of crab into the soup if you like.

Nutrition Facts

Servings: 6

Amount per serving

Calories	268
	% Daily Value*
Total Fat 7.1g	9%
Saturated Fat 1.6g	8%
Cholesterol 134mg	45%
Sodium 285mg	12%
Total Carbohydrate 20.5g	7%
Dietary Fiber 3g	11%
Total Sugars 3.7g	
Protein 31.4g	
Vitamin D 0mcg	1%
Calcium 112mg	9%
Iron 2mg	10%
Potassium 772mg	16%

Diet-related Tips:

- Use red potatoes only if you can tolerate it. If not, simply remove it from the recipe.

BARLEY/OATMEAL SOUP

A delicious Mediterranean soup with healthy, rich ingredients for people with rheumatoid arthritis!

- Prep Time: 10 minutes
- Soak Time: 120 minutes
- Cook Time: 40 minutes
- Total Time: 50 (or 170) minutes
- Serving: 6

Ingredients

- 1 cup barley or oatmeal
- 1 tablespoon gluten-free flour
- 1.5 cup soy or almond milk
- 1 cup carrot, peeled and cubed 1 inch (~2.54 cm)
- 5 cups low-sodium chicken broth

- 1 tablespoon extra virgin olive oil
- 1 tablespoon fresh lemon, squeezed
- Pepper, to taste
- 1 tablespoon parsley, chopped (optional)

Instructions

1. First, let the barley soak for 2 hours. You can use oatmeal if you do not want to wait for 2 hours.
2. In a large pot, cook barley (or oatmeal) and carrots with chicken broth over medium heat for 30 minutes. Add Pepper. Stir occasionally.
3. In a medium pan, make a béchamel sauce: heat extra virgin olive oil. Add flour to the oil and stir until golden brown. Slowly add warm milk to the pan and stir perfectly until thickened. If the sauce is very thick, add more milk.
4. Add béchamel sauce to the pot and add lemon juice. Stir well over low heat for 5-10 more minutes.
5. Garnish the top with chopped parsley. Enjoy!

Cooking Tips:

- You may want to add ½ cup skin-removed chicken breast to your soup to make a chicken-barley soup.
- An orange-color barley soup can be made by one or two tablespoon(s) tomato paste and 1 cup of water instead of 1.5 cups of milk.

Diet-related Tips:

- If you cannot tolerate tomato, do not use the orange version of this soup explained in the cooking tips section.

Nutrition Facts

Servings: 6

Amount per serving	
Calories	**185**
	% Daily Value*
Total Fat 3.7g	5%
Saturated Fat 0.9g	4%
Cholesterol 3mg	1%
Sodium 125mg	5%
Total Carbohydrate 29.8g	11%
Dietary Fiber 5.9g	21%
Total Sugars 4.4g	
Protein 8.5g	
Vitamin D 32mcg	159%
Calcium 89mg	7%
Iron 2mg	9%
Potassium 293mg	6%

HOMEMADE VEGETABLE BROTH

It is an excellent idea for people with rheumatoid arthritis to make their homemade vegetable broth instead of purchasing it from the stores. Many vegetable products are high in sodium and are mixed vegetables that cannot be well-tolerated by some people with rheumatoid arthritis.

- Prep Time: 10 minutes
- Cook Time: 45 minutes
- Total Time: 55 minutes
- Serving: 4-6

<u>Ingredients</u>

- 4 cups celery, chopped
- 4 cups carrot, skin-removed and cubed
- 4 cups of water
- 2 tablespoons fresh lemon juice
- 2 tablespoons extra virgin olive oil
- ½ tablespoon turmeric powder
- 1 bay leaf
- 1 tablespoon fresh parsley, chopped
- ½ teaspoon pepper

<u>Instructions</u>

1. Choose a large pan and cook vegetables with extra virgin olive oil, turmeric powder, and pepper over medium heat until golden brown.
2. Put ingredients in the pan into a large pot, add water, lemon juice, bay leaf, and chopped fresh parsley (optional). Thoroughly boil over low heat until all ingredients get soft.
3. Clear the broth by a colander. Serve immediately or pour and store in a suitable bottle for further use.

<u>Cooking Tips:</u>

- You can blend all ingredients to have a smoothened soup instead of broth.

Nutrition Facts

Servings: 4

Amount per serving

Calories	**127**
	% Daily Value*
Total Fat 7.4g	9%
Saturated Fat 1.1g	6%
Cholesterol 0mg	0%
Sodium 1038mg	45%
Total Carbohydrate 14.9g	5%
Dietary Fiber 4.7g	17%
Total Sugars 7g	
Protein 1.8g	
Vitamin D 0mcg	0%
Calcium 90mg	7%
Iron 1mg	6%
Potassium 650mg	14%

RUSSIAN CHICKEN SOUP

A great, easy to cook Russian soup for cold winters. Great ingredients for people with rheumatoid arthritis!

- Prep Time: 10 minutes
- Cook Time: 30 minutes
- Total Time: 40 minutes

- Serving: 6

<u>Ingredients</u>

- 3 lbs organic, grass-fed chicken breasts, cubed 1 inch (~2.54 cm)
- ¾ cup Capellini or gluten-free pasta
- 4 cups low-sodium chicken or vegetable broth, or water
- 1 tablespoon extra virgin olive oil
- 1 carrot, skin-removed and cubed 1 inch (~2.54 cm)
- 3 medium red or purple potatoes, cubed & peeled 1 inch (~2.54 cm)
- 2 tablespoons fresh lemon juice
- 1 bay leaf
- Pepper, to taste

<u>Instructions</u>

1. Put all ingredients (except lemon juice and carrot) in a large pot and let it simmer over medium heat for 25 minutes.
2. Add carrots and lemon juice to the soup. Cook it for five more minutes. Then, adjust Pepper as desired.
3. Enjoy!

<u>Cooking Tips:</u>

- If you are in remission, you can fry chicken and carrot in a pan by one tablespoon of extra virgin olive oil and 1-teaspoon turmeric powder until golden brown. Then add chicken and carrot to the soup.

<u>Diet-related Tips:</u>

- Use red potatoes only if you can tolerate it. If not, simply remove it from the recipe.

Nutrition Facts

Servings: 6

Amount per serving

Calories	276
	% Daily Value*
Total Fat 5g	6%
Saturated Fat 1.1g	5%
Cholesterol 66mg	22%
Sodium 70mg	3%
Total Carbohydrate 32.4g	12%
Dietary Fiber 3.8g	13%
Total Sugars 2.2g	
Protein 24.6g	
Vitamin D 0mcg	0%
Calcium 35mg	3%
Iron 2mg	11%
Potassium 779mg	17%

BABA GHANOUSH

A great vegetarian middle-eastern appetizer! You can serve Baba Ghanoush, hot or cold.

- Prep Time: 25 minutes
- Cook Time: 40 minutes
- Total Time: 65 minutes
- Serving: 4-6

Ingredients

- 2 eggplants, skin removed
- ¼ cup tahini
- 1 teaspoon extra virgin olive oil
- ½ tablespoon freshly squeezed lemon juice
- ¼ teaspoon cumin powder
- 1 tablespoon fresh parsley, chopped (optional)

Instructions

1. Place eggplants, cut thin lengthwise into a baking sheet with olive oil. Prick all surfaces with a fork. Broil all sides until it gets golden brown and smell smoky.
2. Turn off the broiler. Heat eggplants in the oven in a 375 °F. Let the eggplants roast for 30 minutes.
3. Remove eggplants from the oven. Cool down for 10 minutes and then add the tahini, lemon juice, and cumin powder to it.
4. Mash the roasted mix with a fork until getting a great smooth texture.
5. Drizzle a little bit of olive oil and fresh parsley on top. Enjoy!

<u>Cooking Tips:</u>

- You can use roasted zucchini instead of the eggplants as well if you cannot consume eggplants.

<u>Diet-related Tips:</u>

- Use this recipe only if you can tolerate nightshades and only during remissions.
- If you are fine with eggplants, it is better to use the eggplants with no seeds/fewer seeds.

Nutrition Facts

Servings: 4

Amount per serving

Calories 168

% Daily Value*

Total Fat 9.8g	13%
Saturated Fat 1.3g	7%
Cholesterol 0mg	0%
Sodium 170mg	7%
Total Carbohydrate 19.4g	7%
Dietary Fiber 11.1g	40%
Total Sugars 8.3g	
Protein 5.3g	
Vitamin D 0mcg	0%
Calcium 90mg	7%
Iron 2mg	11%
Potassium 693mg	15%

SALMON BRUSCHETTA

Experience great tastes of salmon and bread!

- Prep Time: 10 minutes
- Cook Time: 30 minutes
- Total Time: 40 minutes
- Serving: 4

Ingredients

- ½ cup smoked salmon, thinly sliced
- 8 baguette slices or gluten-free bread/baguette
- 1 tablespoon grated horseradish
- 1 tablespoon fresh lemon juice
- 1 tablespoon extra virgin olive oil
- 1 cup Persian cucumbers, peeled & chopped
- 1 teaspoon lemon zest

Instructions

1. Cut your baguette to have 1-inch (~2.54 cm) pieces. Then, toast your baguette pieces.
2. Mix horseradish, olive oil, lemon juice, and zest in a bowl. Grate cucumbers in it.

3. Spread your mix on toast slices and put smoked salmon on top. Enjoy!

<u>Cooking Tips:</u>

- You can use toasts instead of baguette to have a delicious cold sandwich.

Nutrition Facts
Servings: 4

Amount per serving

Calories 224

% Daily Value*

Total Fat 14.8g	19%
Saturated Fat 7.2g	36%
Cholesterol 36mg	12%
Sodium 388mg	17%
Total Carbohydrate 14.9g	5%
Dietary Fiber 0.8g	3%
Total Sugars 1.1g	
Protein 8.2g	
Vitamin D 0mcg	0%
Calcium 38mg	3%
Iron 1mg	8%
Potassium 110mg	2%

GUACAMOLE-LIKE APPETIZER

A modified guacamole recipe for people with rheumatoid arthritis.

- Prep Time: 5 minutes
- Cook Time: 0 minutes
- Total Time: 5 minutes
- Serving: 4-6

<u>Ingredients</u>

- 6 avocados, peeled
- ½ tablespoon extra virgin olive oil
- ¼ cup chopped fresh cilantro
- 2 tablespoons fresh lime juice
- 1 teaspoon fresh lemon juice

<u>Instructions</u>

1- In a large bowl, mash avocados.
2- Add extra virgin olive oil and other ingredients into it.
3- Enjoy!

<u>Cooking Tips:</u>

- You can serve guacamole with tacos if you can tolerate it.

<u>Diet-related Tips:</u>

- If you can tolerate tomatoes and onions (in small amounts), cube, and add them into your guacamole.

Nutrition Facts

Servings: 6

Amount per serving

Calories	422
	% Daily Value*
Total Fat 40.4g	52%
Saturated Fat 8.4g	42%
Cholesterol 0mg	0%
Sodium 207mg	9%
Total Carbohydrate 18g	7%
Dietary Fiber 13.5g	48%
Total Sugars 1.2g	
Protein 3.9g	
Vitamin D 0mcg	0%
Calcium 26mg	2%
Iron 1mg	7%
Potassium 988mg	21%

HOMEMADE LEBANESE HUMMUS

A healthy and tasty middle-eastern appetizer. An excellent option for vegetarians and for people with rheumatoid arthritis in remission.

- Prep Time: 5 minutes
- Cook Time: 60 minutes
- Total Time: 65 minutes

- Serving: 4

Ingredients

- ¼ lb dried chickpeas (soaked in water for one night)
- 1½ tablespoons tahini
- 1 tablespoon lemon juice
- 2 tablespoons extra virgin olive oil, divided
- ¼ teaspoon cumin
- 1 tablespoon water
- 1 teaspoon baking soda (optional)
- 1 teaspoon paprika powder

Instructions

1- First, people with rheumatoid arthritis need to soak the chickpeas overnight in water and optionally add baking soda to the water.
2- Cook your chickpeas in a large pot with water over medium heat for about 1 hour. Check if chickpeas cooked well by crushing one of them with a fork in your hand.
3- When chickpeas cooked, drain them and put them in a blender.
4- Add 1 tablespoon of extra virgin olive oil, lemon juice, tahini, and cumin powder to the blender. Blend until your hummus gets a soft, creamy texture equally.
5- Sprinkle with 1 tablespoon extra virgin olive oil or paprika powder (optional).
6- Serve immediately or fridge it.

Cooking Tips:

- Hummus is well-matched with white pita bread.
- You can serve hummus, hot or cold.

<u>Diet-related Tips:</u>

- Eat hummus in moderation when you are in flare-up.

Nutrition Facts
Servings: 4

Amount per serving
Calories   **198**

	% Daily Value*
Total Fat 11.8g	15%
Saturated Fat 1.6g	8%
Cholesterol 0mg	0%
Sodium 305mg	13%
Total Carbohydrate 18.5g	7%
Dietary Fiber 5.5g	20%
Total Sugars 3.1g	
Protein 6.5g	
Vitamin D 0mcg	0%
Calcium 56mg	4%
Iron 2mg	13%
Potassium 279mg	6%

CRAB DIP WITH WONTON CHIPS

A great, easy-to-make appetizer with crabs in wonton wrappers!

- Prep Time: 5 minutes
- Cook Time: 30 minutes
- Total Time: 35 minutes
- Serving: 6

<u>Ingredients</u>

- 1 package Wonton wrappers or gluten-free wonton wrappers
- 1 teaspoon extra virgin olive oil
- 1 can crab meat, chopped
- ½ cup organic low-sodium low-fat mayonnaise
- 1 tablespoon soy sauce
- ½ teaspoon lemon juice
- 1 scallion, chopped
- 1 tablespoon honey or maple syrup

- ½ teaspoon black pepper

Instructions

1- Preheat oven to 400 °F.
2- Mix all ingredients into a large mixing bowl. Stir well.
3- In a baking dish, pour all the mix and bake for 30 minutes until you see edge bubbles.
4- Diagonally cut wonton wrappers in half and make triangles. Alternatively, you can make wonton cups.
5- Pour the cups with your mix.
6- Spray extra virgin olive oil on a baking sheet. Put triangles on it and spray olive oil on wontons as well. Let the wontons bake for 7 minutes until golden brown.
7- Remove from the oven. Serve and Enjoy!

Cooking Tips:

- You need to watch wontons while baking carefully. They can be burnt fast.
- You can have one teaspoon of stevia instead of honey or maple syrup if you cannot tolerate them.

Diet-related Tips:

- During a flare-up, boil scallion first and then add it to the mix.

Shrimp Salad

Are you looking for a delicious salad with shrimp? You can follow this recipe to have one!

- Prep Time: 5 minutes
- Cook Time: 15 minutes
- Total Time: 20 minutes
- Serving: 2-4

Ingredients

- 1 lb shrimp, peeled
- 1 celery stalk, chopped
- 1 tablespoon extra virgin olive oil
- 1 tablespoon fresh lemon juice
- ½ teaspoon turmeric powder
- Pepper, to taste
- 2 tablespoons organic low-fat low-sodium mayonnaise (optional)

Instructions

1. Cook shrimps by extra virgin olive oil and turmeric in a medium pan over medium heat.

2. In a large bowl, mix all lemon juice, pepper, and mayonnaise (optional).
3. Add cooked shrimp to the bowl and combine.
4. Serve and enjoy!

<u>Cooking Tips:</u>

- You can prepare your shrimps in the oven as well. Just preheat oven to 375 °F. Choose a cooking sheet and spray olive oil on it. Put shrimp on your cooking sheet and let it cook until golden brown (around 10 minutes).

<u>Diet-related Tips:</u>

- Do not use mayonnaise a lot if you are experiencing a flare-up.

Nutrition Facts

Servings: 4

Amount per serving

Calories	197
	% Daily Value*
Total Fat 8g	10%
Saturated Fat 1.5g	7%
Cholesterol 241mg	80%
Sodium 347mg	15%
Total Carbohydrate 3.9g	1%
Dietary Fiber 0.2g	1%
Total Sugars 0.6g	
Protein 26g	
Vitamin D 0mcg	0%
Calcium 107mg	8%
Iron 1mg	3%
Potassium 217mg	5%

Zucchini Salad (Spiralized)

A great summer salad based on a zucchini. Zucchini salad is a healthy choice for people with rheumatoid arthritis.

- Prep Time: 30 minutes
- Total Time: 30 minutes

- Serving: 2-4

Ingredients

- 2 zucchinis, chopped
- 1 tablespoon extra virgin olive oil
- 2 tablespoons fresh lemon juice
- 1 tablespoon parsley, chopped (optional)
- Pepper, to taste

Instructions

1. Make spiral zucchinis or cut them thin and lengthwise
2. In a large bowl, mix zucchinis and all other ingredients.
3. For better taste, let it rest for 15 minutes. Enjoy!

Cooking Tips:

- You can use vegetable peelers if you do not have a spiralizer.

Diet-related Tips:

- Use this recipe if you can tolerate zucchini.
- Boil spiralized zucchini if you are in a flare.

Nutrition Facts

Servings: 4

Amount per serving

Calories 65

% Daily Value*

Total Fat 3.7g	5%
Saturated Fat 0.6g	3%
Cholesterol 2mg	1%
Sodium 141mg	6%
Total Carbohydrate 3.9g	1%
Dietary Fiber 1.1g	4%
Total Sugars 1.9g	
Protein 4.8g	
Vitamin D 0mcg	0%
Calcium 65mg	5%
Iron 0mg	2%
Potassium 266mg	6%

APPLE-PEAR SALAD

A simple great fruit salad for everyone!

- Prep Time: 10 minutes
- Total Time: 10 minutes
- Serving: 4-6

Ingredients

- 3 cooked pears, peeled and chopped
- 1 papaya, peeled and chopped
- 3 apples, peeled and chopped
- ¼ cup honey or maple syrup
- 3 tablespoons fresh lemon juice
- ¼ cup fresh mint leaves, chopped (optional)

Instructions

1. Add all your ingredients in a large bowl and mix well.
2. Serve cold. Enjoy!

Cooking Tips:

- Remove honey or maple syrup from ingredients if you cannot tolerate any of them.

Nutrition Facts

Servings: 4

Amount per serving

Calories 278

	% Daily Value*
Total Fat 0.8g	1%
Saturated Fat 0.1g	1%
Cholesterol 0mg	0%
Sodium 13mg	1%
Total Carbohydrate 73.2g	27%
Dietary Fiber 10.4g	37%
Total Sugars 56.5g	
Protein 1.6g	
Vitamin D 0mcg	0%
Calcium 33mg	3%
Iron 1mg	7%
Potassium 529mg	11%

BEET, CARROT & APPLE SALAD

A colorful salad with amazing fruits and vegetables inside!

- Prep Time: 10 minutes
- Total Time: 10 minutes
- Serving: 4-6

Ingredients

- 1 lb beet, peeled and cubed 1 inch (~2.54 cm)
- 2 medium carrots, peeled and cubed 1 inch (~2.54 cm)
- 1 apple, peeled and cubed 1 inch (~2.54 cm)
- 3 tablespoons fresh orange juice
- 2 tablespoons fresh lime juice
- 1 tablespoon extra virgin olive oil
- Pepper, to taste
- ¼ cup fresh mint leaves, chopped (optional)

Instructions

1. In a large bowl, mix well all ingredients.
2. Serve cold. Enjoy!

<u>Cooking Tips:</u>

- Wear gloves to cover your hands when you cut beets.

<u>Diet-related Tips:</u>

- Cook beets well when you are experiencing a flare-up.

Nutrition Facts
Servings: 4

Amount per serving

Calories	129
	% Daily Value*
Total Fat 3.8g	5%
Saturated Fat 0.5g	3%
Cholesterol 0mg	0%
Sodium 109mg	5%
Total Carbohydrate 24.1g	9%
Dietary Fiber 4.4g	16%
Total Sugars 17.5g	
Protein 2.4g	
Vitamin D 0mcg	0%
Calcium 30mg	2%
Iron 1mg	8%
Potassium 539mg	11%

BUTTER LETTUCE SALAD WITH HONEY VINAIGRETTE

A light and delicious salad for people with rheumatoid arthritis who can tolerate butter lettuce with a delicious dressing.

- Prep Time: 15 minutes
- Total Time: 15 minutes
- Serving: 4-6

<u>Ingredients</u>

- 2 medium butter lettuces, cut into small pieces (also called Bibb, Boston or living lettuce)
- 1 tablespoon honey or maple syrup
- 2 tablespoons fresh lemon juice
- 2 tablespoons fresh lime juice

- 2 tablespoons extra virgin olive oil
- Pepper to taste

Instructions

1. Wash butter lettuce thoroughly and cut into small pieces
2. In a large bowl, mix well all ingredients.
3. Serve cold. Enjoy!

Cooking Tips:

- You can add two peeled Persian cucumbers to have a garden-like salad!

Diet-related Tips:

- Butter lettuce, also called Bibb, living or Boston lettuce, is a type of lettuce that can be digested easier than other types of lettuce. Hence, it is an excellent option for people with rheumatoid arthritis who also have gastrointestinal issues such as IBS or IBD. Many people with rheumatoid arthritis can enjoy a garden salad with butter lettuce during remissions.

Nutrition Facts

Servings: 4

Amount per serving

Calories	91
	% Daily Value*
Total Fat 7.1g	9%
Saturated Fat 1.1g	5%
Cholesterol 0mg	0%
Sodium 21mg	1%
Total Carbohydrate 7.5g	3%
Dietary Fiber 1.1g	4%
Total Sugars 5.7g	
Protein 1.2g	
Vitamin D 0mcg	0%
Calcium 33mg	3%
Iron 0mg	1%
Potassium 237mg	5%

Carrot-Avocado Salad

An epic salad recipe with avocado and tasty dressing. A great salad option for people with rheumatoid arthritis!

- Prep Time: 20 minutes
- Cook Time: 30 minutes
- Total Time: 50 minutes
- Serving: 4-6

Ingredients

- 1 large avocado
- 2 carrots, peeled and diced 1-inch (~2.54 cm)
- 2 tablespoons extra virgin olive oil
- 1 tablespoon fresh lemon juice
- Pepper, to taste
- ⅓ cup green onion, chopped
- ¼ cup fresh mint leaves, chopped (optional)

Instructions

1. Peel-off carrots.
2. In a small pot, cook carrots in boiling water over medium heat.
3. Cube carrots and avocados. In a medium bowl, mix other ingredients and then add carrot and avocado.
4. Mix well. Enjoy!

Cooking Tips:

- You can cook carrots in a small pan with one tablespoon of extra virgin olive oil and ½ teaspoon of turmeric powder over medium heat as well.

Nutrition Facts

Servings: 4

Amount per serving

Calories	179
	% Daily Value*
Total Fat 16.9g	22%
Saturated Fat 3.1g	15%
Cholesterol 0mg	0%
Sodium 26mg	1%
Total Carbohydrate 8g	3%
Dietary Fiber 4.4g	16%
Total Sugars 2g	
Protein 1.4g	
Vitamin D 0mcg	0%
Calcium 22mg	2%
Iron 1mg	3%
Potassium 369mg	8%

CLASSIC TUNA PASTA SALAD

Classic tuna with pasta is an excellent choice as your salad. You can have it for lunch or dinner as well.

- Prep Time: 15 minutes
- Cook Time: 15 minutes
- Total Time: 30 minutes
- Serving: 4

<u>Ingredients</u>

- 1½ cups brown rice pasta or gluten-free quinoa pasta
- 1 celery stalk, chopped
- 1 can tuna in water or extra virgin olive oil
- ½ cup organic low-fat low-sodium mayonnaise
- 2 tablespoons lemon juice
- Pepper, to taste

<u>Instructions</u>

1. Cook pasta according to its package instruction.
2. Drain pasta and place it in a large bowl.

3. Add celery, tuna, and all other ingredients to the pasta bowl. Mix well.

4. It is better to let it cool in the fridge for 30 minutes. Enjoy!

Nutrition Facts

Servings: 4

Amount per serving

Calories	105
	% Daily Value*
Total Fat 3g	4%
Saturated Fat 0.7g	3%
Cholesterol 25mg	8%
Sodium 526mg	23%
Total Carbohydrate 8.9g	3%
Dietary Fiber 1.4g	5%
Total Sugars 4.9g	
Protein 10.4g	
Vitamin D 0mcg	0%
Calcium 13mg	1%
Iron 1mg	3%
Potassium 159mg	3%

SALMON CEVICHE

This salad is full of omega-3 with a fabulous dressing. Enjoy this dairy-free, egg-free, nut-free, and gluten-free recipe.

- Prep Time: 15 minutes
- Rest Time: 15 minutes
- Total Time: 30 minutes
- Serving: 4

Ingredients

- 1 lb salmon, skin removed and cubed
- 1 cup Persian cucumber, cubed 1cm
- ½ cup green onion, chopped well
- 1 tablespoon fresh lemon juice
- 1 tablespoon fresh lime juice
- 1 tablespoon grated fresh ginger
- Pepper, to taste

- 1 teaspoon dried oregano (optional)

<u>Instructions</u>

1. In a large bowl, mix salmon, cucumber, green onion, ginger, and oregano.
2. In a small cup/bowl, whisk lime & lemon juice, and pepper and pour it into the large bowl.
3. Mix all well. Serve cold. Enjoy!

<u>Cooking Tips:</u>

- You can add ½ teaspoon freshly grated turmeric if you want to enjoy its anti-inflammatory properties.

Nutrition Facts

Servings: 4

Amount per serving

Calories	167
	% Daily Value*
Total Fat 7.1g	9%
Saturated Fat 1.1g	5%
Cholesterol 50mg	17%
Sodium 53mg	2%
Total Carbohydrate 3.9g	1%
Dietary Fiber 1.1g	4%
Total Sugars 0.6g	
Protein 22.4g	
Vitamin D 0mcg	0%
Calcium 52mg	4%
Iron 1mg	6%
Potassium 506mg	11%

Honey Chicken Salad

Enjoy making a rich salad with chicken and honey. Excellent source of protein for people with rheumatoid arthritis.

- Prep Time: 25 minutes
- Total Time: 25 minutes
- Serving: 4-6

<u>Ingredients</u>

- 1 lb chicken breasts, skinless and boneless
- 1 avocado, chopped
- 4 tablespoons honey or maple syrup (if you can tolerate)
- 6 cups butter lettuce, chopped
- 3 tablespoons lemon juice
- 2 tablespoons extra virgin olive oil
- Pepper, to taste
- 1 tablespoon green onion, chopped (optional)

Instructions

1. In a large pan, cook chickens with two tablespoons of extra virgin olive oil over medium heat until getting close to a golden brown. Remove from pan and cut into 1-inch (~2.54 cm) cubes.
2. In a large bowl, whisk honey (or maple syrup), lemon juice, green onion (optional), and pepper.
3. In another large bowl, cut lettuce into small pieces. Add cubed chickens and pour the sauce on top. Serve and enjoy!

Cooking Tips:

- You can boil chickens in a pot over medium heat (recommended for flare-up times).
- If you cannot tolerate honey, use maple syrup or agave syrup instead.

MAIN COURSES

MEDITERRANEAN CHICKEN - ZUCCHINI STEW

Chicken–Zucchini stew is one of the delicious Mediterranean stews, which can be served with steamed brown rice. Turmeric, zucchini, and brown rice are great for people with rheumatoid arthritis and most can well-tolerate them.

- Prep Time: 10 minutes
- Cook Time: 50 minutes
- Total Time: 60 minutes
- Serving: 4

<u>Ingredients</u>

- 4 Fresh zucchinis, lengthwise-cut with no skin
- 6 Skin-removed chicken legs
- 4 tablespoons extra virgin olive oil
- 1.5 teaspoon turmeric
- ½ teaspoon black pepper
- 3 tablespoons lemon juice or 1 lime
- 2½ cups water

- 4 tablespoons tomato paste (optional)

<u>Preparation</u>

1. Fry, both sides of skinless zucchinis with two tablespoons of extra virgin olive oil in a sauté pan until golden brown.
2. In another pan, fry your chicken legs with the rest of extra virgin olive oil, pepper, and turmeric until golden brown.
3. Boil water in a pot and dissolve tomato paste to the boiling water if you want (optional). Stir well.
4. Add your chicken legs to the boiling water. Turn the heat to medium. Let it simmer for 20 minutes. If your sauce gets thick, add more water to your stew.
5. After 25 minutes, add your zucchinis and your lemon juice to the stew and let it cook for another 5 minutes. After three minutes, taste your stew and correct your seasonings. Do not add more black peppers.
6. Enjoy this meal with steamed brown rice!

<u>Cooking Tips:</u>

- To reach a faster cooking time, you can add all the ingredients into the boiling water and let the stew cook for 40 minutes on high heat.
- You can use eggplant instead of zucchini to make a delicious Eggplant Stew. Just remember not to use the eggplants seeds or remove eggplant small edible seeds.

<u>Diet-related Tips:</u>

- Some patients cannot tolerate tomato pastes. In that case, cook this stew without tomato paste or use two cups of organic vegetable broth instead of water.
- If you are in a flare-up, remove zucchini's skins.
- Use this recipe only if you can tolerate nightshades such as zucchini.

Nutrition Facts

Servings: 4

Amount per serving

Calories	352
	% Daily Value*
Total Fat 22.6g	29%
Saturated Fat 4.4g	22%
Cholesterol 89mg	30%
Sodium 1001mg	44%
Total Carbohydrate 10.5g	4%
Dietary Fiber 3.1g	11%
Total Sugars 5.6g	
Protein 28.9g	
Vitamin D 0mcg	0%
Calcium 55mg	4%
Iron 3mg	16%
Potassium 945mg	20%

CHICKEN FETTUCCINE ALFREDO

Do you love to have a creamy-but-healthy Fettuccine Alfredo? You can use this recipe to have a delicious Italian main course. This meal has chicken/vegetable stock, turmeric, ginger, and lemon that are great for people with rheumatoid arthritis.

- Prep Time: 15 minutes
- Cook Time: 30 minutes
- Total Time: 45 minutes
- Serving: 4

<u>Ingredients</u>

- 4 boneless, skinless chicken breasts, about 0.8 inches (~2 cm) thick

- ¾ lb (~340 g) uncooked brown rice fettucine or gluten-free fettuccine/pasta
- 3 tablespoons gluten-free flour
- 10 oz almond milk (~300 ml)
- ½ cup unsalted organic chicken stock or vegetable stock (~120 ml)
- 1 tablespoon fresh lemon juice
- 2 teaspoons black pepper, divided
- 1 teaspoon turmeric
- 1 teaspoon ginger powder
- 3 tablespoons extra virgin olive oil, divided
- Fresh parsley, minced (optional)

<u>Preparation</u>

1. Heat a tablespoon of extra virgin olive oil in a pan. Add your chicken breast with one tablespoon of pepper and turmeric and let it cook for 5 minutes until golden brown both sides.
2. Boil the water in a large pot over high heat. Add one tablespoon of high-quality extra virgin olive oil to the water. Then, add your fettuccine in the boiling water.
3. Cook fettuccine according to its package instructions. Drain and return to the pot.
4. In another pan, put one tablespoon of extra virgin olive oil on medium heat. When heated, add your flour slowly and whisk until golden brown.
5. Heat your milk in the microwave, add it slowly to your flour, and whisk for 3 minutes. Add lemon juice, ginger powder, and one tablespoon of pepper to make an excellent béchamel sauce.
6. Add chicken/vegetable stock to the béchamel sauce, frequently stir for 10 minutes until thickened.

7. Slice or cube chicken. Add the béchamel sauce to your fettuccine pot and toss perfectly.

8. Garnish the top with minced parsley and enjoy!

<u>Cooking Tips:</u>

- If you are gluten intolerant, you have to use gluten-free pasta/fettuccine.

<u>Diet-related Tips:</u>

- Make sure that your chickens are skinless.

Nutrition Facts

Servings: 4

Amount per serving

Calories	626
	% Daily Value*
Total Fat 23.2g	30%
Saturated Fat 5.1g	25%
Cholesterol 170mg	57%
Sodium 2433mg	106%
Total Carbohydrate 51g	19%
Dietary Fiber 3.6g	13%
Total Sugars 1.3g	
Protein 50.5g	
Vitamin D 0mcg	0%
Calcium 52mg	4%
Iron 4mg	20%
Potassium 387mg	8%

CHICKEN STROGANOFF

Try Chicken Stroganoff with red/purple potatoes and incredible gravy, matched with patient's tolerance levels.

- Prep Time: 5 minutes
- Cook Time: 15 minutes
- Total Time: 20 minutes
- Serving: 4

<u>Ingredients</u>

- 4 skinless, boneless chicken breast

- 2 tablespoons gluten-free flour
- 2 cups (~500 ml) unsalted/salt-reduced chicken broth (organic preferred)
- 1 tablespoon pepper
- 3 tablespoons extra virgin olive oil
- ⅓ cup almond or soy milk
- 1 tablespoon fresh lemon juice
- ½ tablespoon ginger powder or fresh ginger
- ½ tablespoon turmeric
- 10 oz (~300 gr) mushrooms, thickly sliced
- Parsley, minced (optional)

Instructions

1. Heat a tablespoon of high-quality extra virgin olive oil in a pan. Flat your chicken breasts and cook them with ½ tablespoon of pepper and ginger powder until golden brown both sides.
2. In another pan, put one tablespoon of extra virgin olive oil on medium heat. When heated, sauté your mushrooms. Then, add your flour slowly and whisk until golden brown.
3. Heat your milk in the microwave, add it slowly to your flour, and whisk for 3 minutes. Add lemon juice, and ½ tablespoon of pepper to make a great sauce. Stir the sauce on low heat until it becomes thick.
4. Fry very thin-sliced potatoes with one tablespoon of extra virgin olive oil and ½ tablespoon of turmeric.
5. Add your fries and chicken to your sauce. Let it cook for two more minutes.
6. Garnish the top with minced parsley and enjoy!

Cooking Tips:

- You can use pork tenderloin or turkey breast instead of chicken breast.

Diet-related Tips:

- Make sure that your chickens and red/purple potatoes are skinless.
- If you are in a flare-up, try to Airfry your fries or boil them.
- If you cannot use potatoes, you can serve the chicken with gluten-free pasta such as brown rice or quinoa.

Nutrition Facts

Servings: 4

Amount per serving

Calories	**274**
	% Daily Value*
Total Fat 13.2g	17%
Saturated Fat 1.9g	10%
Cholesterol 67mg	22%
Sodium 433mg	19%
Total Carbohydrate 10.7g	4%
Dietary Fiber 2.6g	9%
Total Sugars 2.7g	
Protein 29.8g	
Vitamin D 15mcg	77%
Calcium 42mg	3%
Iron 3mg	17%
Potassium 331mg	7%

CHICKEN KEBAB

Enjoy a classic barbecued chicken, well-marinated in saffron and yogurt!

- Prep Time: 15 minutes
- (Marinate Time: 2 hours)
- Cook Time: 25 minutes
- Total Time: 40 minutes
- Serving: 4

Ingredients

- 4 chicken breasts, cut into 1.5 inches (3.8) cubes
- ¾ cup lactose-free yogurt or plain yogurt if you are not lactose intolerant
- 1 large onion
- ¼ cup saffron (bloomed)
- 3 tablespoons extra virgin olive oil
- 1 tablespoon lemon juice

Instructions

1. Cut your onions and make onion rings.
2. To marinate your chicken, mix and stir it well with onion, lactose-free plain yogurt, bloomed saffron, olive oil, and lemon juice together (To have a bloomed saffron, you need to grind your saffron perfectly and add 100ml of boiling water to it).
3. Cover the marinated bowl and put it in the fridge to rest for two hours.
4. After two hours, thread chickens into skewers and grilled both sides well until golden brown

Cooking Tips:

- If you are not lactose-intolerant, you can use low-fat plain yogurt.
- You can use the oven instead of grilling chickens. Just preheat the oven to 400 °F, cover chickens with aluminum foils, and let it cook for about 25 minutes. Use broil for five minutes if you want a golden brown texture.
- You can use chicken with bones instead of chicken breasts, as well.

Diet-related Tips:

- If you cannot tolerate saffron (rarely happens), do not add it to the mix. Instead, put ⅓ tablespoon of turmeric.

Nutrition Facts

Servings: 4

Amount per serving

Calories	322
	% Daily Value*
Total Fat 21g	27%
Saturated Fat 2.5g	12%
Cholesterol 68mg	23%
Sodium 1812mg	79%
Total Carbohydrate 7.4g	3%
Dietary Fiber 0.9g	3%
Total Sugars 1.7g	
Protein 27.6g	
Vitamin D 0mcg	0%
Calcium 70mg	5%
Iron 0mg	2%
Potassium 174mg	4%

CHICKEN WITH POMEGRANATE SAUCE

Have you tried a sour taste of chicken with pomegranate sauce? This dish is an excellent sample of a delicious sour chicken. You can make your dish sweet and sour by adding honey to the recipe.

- Prep Time: 10 minutes
- (Marinate Time: 2 hours)
- Cook Time: 40 minutes
- Total Time: 50 minutes
- Serving: 4

Ingredients

- 4 Chicken legs and thighs, skinless
- ¼ cup bloomed saffron
- 2 tablespoons extra virgin olive oil
- 5 tablespoons lime juice
- ½ cup pomegranate sauce
- 1 tablespoon turmeric

- 2 cups of water
- ½ tablespoon Black pepper
- ½ cup honey (optional)

Instructions

1. In a large bowl, marinate your chicken with bloomed saffron, lime juice, honey (optional), and pepper.
2. Mix and stir all ingredients well. Cover the bowl top and fridge it for 2 hours.
3. Roast your chicken with extra virgin olive oil and turmeric for 15 minutes until golden brown.
4. Boil two cups of water and add pomegranate sauce. Stir well until dissolved.
5. Put your chicken in the sauce and let it cook for 25 minutes. Let the sauce thicken, and then you are done!
6. Serve it with white basmati rice and enjoy!

Cooking Tips:

- Alternatively, you may want to use chicken breasts instead of chicken legs and thighs.
- If you do not find the pomegranate sauce or paste, you can add 200ml of pomegranate juice. It makes your meal hard to be thickened, but it gives you a similar taste.

Diet-related Tips:

- If you cannot tolerate saffron (rarely happens), do not add saffron to chicken. Instead, put ⅓ tablespoon of turmeric.
- Pomegranate has anti-inflammatory properties, which is excellent for people with rheumatoid

arthritis and it can be well-tolerate by many patients. However, if you cannot tolerate it, use dark grape juice instead. Make sure pomegranates are consumed seedless.

Nutrition Facts

Servings: 4

Amount per serving

Calories   **303**

	% Daily Value*
Total Fat 17.2g	22%
Saturated Fat 3.6g	18%
Cholesterol 90mg	30%
Sodium 2094mg	91%
Total Carbohydrate 16.4g	6%
Dietary Fiber 0.6g	2%
Total Sugars 11.4g	
Protein 22.7g	
Vitamin D 0mcg	0%
Calcium 33mg	3%
Iron 2mg	13%
Potassium 79mg	2%

PUFFY CHICKEN

A tremendous yummy puffy chicken strips for adults and kids.

- Prep Time: 10 minutes
- Cook Time: 20 minutes
- Total Time: 30 minutes
- Serving: 4

<u>Ingredients</u>

- 4 strip cuts of chicken breast (~400 grams)
- 150 grams of gluten-free flour such as almond flour
- 5 tablespoons alcohol-free carbonated malt drink
- 2 tablespoons extra virgin olive oil
- 3 eggs (organic range-free preferred)
- ½ tablespoon turmeric powder
- ½ teaspoon stevia or maple syrup (optional)
- 1 tablespoon active dried yeast (optional)

<u>Instructions</u>

1. In a large bowl, marinate your chicken with malt drink, yeast, olive oil, and turmeric. Mix all well.
2. In another bowl, whisk all three eggs perfectly.
3. First, deep your marinated chickens into eggs and then cover it with flour.
4. Cook your chicken in a pan over medium heat with extra virgin olive oil.

<u>Cooking Tips:</u>

- You can use stevia or maple syrup to give a sweet taste to your dish.
- Instead of carbonated malt drink, you can use carbonated water. In this case, you need to use active dry yeast.

<u>Diet-related Tips:</u>

- If you are in a flare-up, put your marinated chicken in boiling water instead of frying it.

Nutrition Facts

Servings: 4

Amount per serving	
Calories	**458**
	% Daily Value*
Total Fat 16g	20%
Saturated Fat 3.5g	18%
Cholesterol 221mg	74%
Sodium 1051mg	46%
Total Carbohydrate 31.8g	12%
Dietary Fiber 1.3g	5%
Total Sugars 2g	
Protein 44.3g	
Vitamin D 12mcg	58%
Calcium 46mg	4%
Iron 4mg	22%
Potassium 410mg	9%

CHICKEN SCALOPPINI

Enjoy a delicious Italian dish with ingredients great for people with rheumatoid arthritis!

- Prep Time: 10 minutes
- Cook Time: 15 minutes
- Total Time: 25 minutes
- Serving: 4

Ingredients

- 4 skinless and boneless chicken breast
- 2 teaspoons fresh lemon juice
- 1 tablespoon extra virgin olive oil
- 6 tablespoons wholegrain bread crumbs or any gluten-free dried bread
- ½ cup unsalted, no-fat chicken broth
- 1 tablespoon lime juice
- 1 tablespoon well-cooked capers
- ¼ teaspoon black pepper

Instructions

1. First, use a meat mallet to pound your chicken breasts.
2. Add lemon juice, and pepper to your chicken
3. Heat a pan with extra virgin olive oil over medium heat. Add your chicken to the pan and cook each side for about 5 minutes until golden brown.
4. In the end, add chicken broth and your breadcrumbs and stir well for five more minutes until it gets thick.
5. Garnish with capers. Enjoy!

Diet-related Tips:

- Make sure you cooked capers well.

- If you are in a flare-up, do not need to fry chicken. Just boil it in chicken broth.

Nutrition Facts

Servings: 4

Amount per serving	
Calories	**320**
	% Daily Value*
Total Fat 11g	14%
Saturated Fat 2.6g	13%
Cholesterol 35mg	12%
Sodium 863mg	38%
Total Carbohydrate 33.2g	12%
Dietary Fiber 1.5g	6%
Total Sugars 0.7g	
Protein 20.6g	
Vitamin D 0mcg	0%
Calcium 19mg	1%
Iron 2mg	9%
Potassium 28mg	1%

CHICKEN PIZZA

Do you think lactose-intolerant patients cannot eat pizza anymore? You might be wrong! Try this recipe to have a great pizza taste!

- Prep Time: 10 minutes
- Cook Time: 15 minutes
- Total Time: 25 minutes
- Serving: 4

Ingredients

- 4 gluten-free pizza crusts
- 1 cup sliced no-fat cooked chicken breast
- 1 cup lactose-free plant-based dairy-free cheese
- 4 tablespoons organic low-sodium mayonnaise
- 1 teaspoon oregano powder

Instructions

1. Place your gluten-free pizza crusts on a non-stick pizza pan or bake sheet.
2. Spread your organic low-fat low-sodium mayo on your crust.
3. Add your cooked chicken breasts to your pizza
4. Sprinkle with lactose-free plant-based cheese
5. Let it bake at 480 °F for 10 minutes. Then, broil on the same heat for five more minutes until cheese melted.

<u>Cooking Tips:</u>

- You can use any other white sauces such as béchamel sauce instead of mayo.

<u>Diet-related Tips:</u>

- Use mayonnaise only if you can tolerate it. If you cannot tolerate, you can make a béchamel sauce instead (explained before in Fettuccine Alfredo recipe).

Nutrition Facts

Servings: 4

Amount per serving

Calories	342
	% Daily Value*
Total Fat 12.4g	16%
Saturated Fat 2.7g	14%
Cholesterol 47mg	16%
Sodium 499mg	22%
Total Carbohydrate 39.1g	14%
Dietary Fiber 2.1g	7%
Total Sugars 7g	
Protein 18.5g	
Vitamin D 0mcg	0%
Calcium 82mg	6%
Iron 1mg	7%
Potassium 165mg	4%

TURKEY ZUCCHINI NOODLES

If you look for a healthy meal for your lunch or dinner, you can try Turkey Zucchini Noodles. If you have some leftover turkeys from Thanksgiving or any other events, it would be an excellent option for you to cook this delicious main course.

- Prep Time: 15 minutes
- Cook Time: 15 minutes
- Total Time: 30 minutes
- Serving: 4

<u>Ingredients</u>

- 3 medium-size spiralized zucchinis or zucchini strips
- 1 lb (~455 g) skinless fat-free cooked turkey breasts
- 1 tablespoon extra virgin olive oil, divided
- 2 cups of water
- ½ teaspoon turmeric
- 1 tablespoon tomato paste (optional)
- ¼ teaspoon stevia (optional)

<u>Instructions</u>

1. Cook zucchini noodles in boiling water for 5 minutes.
2. Bring them out of the water and let them dry.
3. Heat your cooked turkey in a pan with extra virgin olive oil. Add turmeric, tomato paste (optional), stevia (optional), and little water (~100ml) for 5 minutes until golden brown both sides.
4. Add your zucchini to your turkey and stir well. Enjoy!

<u>Cooking Tips:</u>

- You can use a can of organic crushed tomatoes instead of tomato paste if you can tolerate them.

<u>Diet-related Tips:</u>

- If you are in a flare-up, do not need to golden-brown turkey. Just boil it in 1 cup of zucchini water.
- Use zucchini and tomato paste only if you can tolerate it.

Nutrition Facts

Servings: 4

Amount per serving

Calories	172
	% Daily Value*
Total Fat 5.7g	7%
Saturated Fat 0.9g	5%
Cholesterol 49mg	16%
Sodium 1460mg	63%
Total Carbohydrate 9.9g	4%
Dietary Fiber 2.3g	8%
Total Sugars 6.5g	
Protein 21.2g	
Vitamin D 0mcg	0%
Calcium 35mg	3%
Iron 2mg	13%
Potassium 736mg	16%

ZUCCHINI EGG DISH

Are you looking for a vegetarian dish that is well-matched with RA anti-inflammatory diet? Try a fabulous Zucchini Egg dish.

- Prep Time: 10 minutes
- Cook Time: 15 minutes
- Total Time: 25 minutes
- Serving: 4

<u>Ingredients</u>

- 3 medium-size, diced zucchinis
- 2 organic range-free eggs
- 1 tablespoon extra virgin olive oil
- ½ teaspoon turmeric powder
- ½ teaspoon black pepper

<u>Instructions</u>

1. Peels off zucchinis and cook them in a pan over medium heat.
2. When zucchinis become soft, flattened them or blend them in a blender.
3. Add turmeric, and pepper to your pan.
4. Whisk eggs in a small bowl and add them to your zucchinis.
5. When the eggs get coagulate, mix them with your zucchinis. Enjoy!

Cooking Tips:

- You can use eggplant instead of zucchini only if you can tolerate eggplant.
- You can also add one tablespoon of tomato paste if you can tolerate it.

Diet-related Tips:

- If you are in a flare-up, do not need to fry zucchinis. Just boil them in 1 cup of water.
- Use this recipe only if you can tolerate zucchini.

Nutrition Facts

Servings: 4

Amount per serving

Calories	94
	% Daily Value*
Total Fat 6g	8%
Saturated Fat 1.2g	6%
Cholesterol 82mg	27%
Sodium 337mg	15%
Total Carbohydrate 7g	3%
Dietary Fiber 2g	7%
Total Sugars 3.2g	
Protein 5g	
Vitamin D 8mcg	39%
Calcium 37mg	3%
Iron 1mg	7%
Potassium 448mg	10%

GINGER STICKY PORK

Are you looking for a satisfying, easy to cook a meal with pork? Ginger Sticky Pork is a great candidate for you and your family members who is on an RA diet.

- Prep Time: 15 minutes
- Cook Time: 10 minutes
- Total Time: 25 minutes
- Serving: 6

Ingredients

- 1½ lb boneless, fat-removed pork tenderloin, cut into strips with ½ inch (~1.3cm) thickness
- 1 tablespoon extra virgin olive oil
- ½ cup honey or maple syrup
- 2 inches (~5cm) fresh ginger knob
- 1 tablespoon lemon juice
- ½ teaspoon black pepper

Instructions

1. Heat extra virgin olive oil in a skillet over medium-high heat until shimmering.
2. Add your pork and pepper to the skillet. Brown one side first and then brown the other side of pork. Take out your pork.
3. Add ginger, lemon juice, and honey to the pan. Stir and bring to boil.
4. When the sauce gets thick and sticky like honey, bring back your pork. Enjoy!

Cooking Tips:

- This dish can be served perfectly with steamed brown rice.

<u>Diet-related Tips:</u>

- Boil pork in water if you are in a severe flare-up. Then, take the pork out of boiling water and add them to your sticky sauce.
- If you cannot use honey, you can use maple syrup, ½ teaspoon of stevia or agave syrup.

Nutrition Facts

Servings: 6

Amount per serving	
Calories	**275**
	% Daily Value*
Total Fat 6.4g	8%
Saturated Fat 1.7g	9%
Cholesterol 83mg	28%
Sodium 454mg	20%
Total Carbohydrate 24.9g	9%
Dietary Fiber 0.4g	1%
Total Sugars 23.5g	
Protein 30g	
Vitamin D 0mcg	0%
Calcium 12mg	1%
Iron 2mg	9%
Potassium 521mg	11%

German Pork Schnitzel

If you are looking for tender pork with a crispy crust, try German Pork Schnitzel. It is very easy to make it, and it is well-matched with baby carrots as a garnish.

- Prep Time: 20 minutes
- Cook Time: 15 minutes
- Total Time: 35 minutes
- Serving: 4

<u>Ingredients</u>

- 2 lbs boneless fatless pork tenderloins flattened into ½ inch (1.3cm) thick
- 3 large organic free-range eggs

- 2 cups wholegrain bread crumbs or gluten-free bread crumbs
- ⅓ cup gluten-free flour such as almond flour
- 2 tablespoons extra virgin olive oil
- Lemon wedges for taste
- ½ teaspoon black pepper

<u>Instructions</u>

1. Pound your pork pieces with a mallet until it gets ½ inch thick.
2. In a medium bowl, mix flour, and pepper.
3. In another bowl, whisk three eggs.
4. In another bowl or plate, spread your breadcrumbs.
5. First, put both sides of pork cutlets in flour. Then, dip them in egg and then drip them into breadcrumbs using a fork.
6. Now, heat a large pan with extra virgin olive oil over medium heat. When the oil gets very hot, cook your cutlets for 5 minutes, each side until each side gets golden brown.
7. Enjoy the meal with lemon wedges!

<u>Cooking Tips:</u>

- Use gluten-free bread crumbs and flour if you are gluten intolerant.

<u>Diet-related Tips:</u>

- Use only one egg if you cannot tolerate eggs well during a flare-up.
- During remission, do not stir fry your schnitzel at all. Just spray 2 tablespoons of extra virgin olive oil and fry it.

Nutrition Facts

Servings: 4

Amount per serving	
Calories	**600**

	% Daily Value*
Total Fat 19.3g	25%
Saturated Fat 4.7g	23%
Cholesterol 243mg	81%
Sodium 979mg	43%
Total Carbohydrate 49.6g	18%
Dietary Fiber 2.9g	10%
Total Sugars 5.7g	
Protein 54.5g	
Vitamin D 12mcg	58%
Calcium 120mg	9%
Iron 6mg	33%
Potassium 169mg	4%

BAKED APPLE PORK

A delicious pork-based recipe that has been modified for people with rheumatoid arthritis.

- Prep Time: 5 minutes
- Cook Time: 35 minutes
- Total Time: 40 minutes
- Serving: 4

Ingredients

- 2 lbs skinless, boneless pork tenderloin
- 1 cup large apple, cut into small cubes
- 1 tablespoon peeled and grated ginger (~1 inch or ~2.5 cm)
- 2 tablespoons soy sauce
- 2 tablespoons extra virgin olive oil
- Black pepper, to taste

Instructions

1. Mix ginger, balsamic, and soy sauce in a small bowl.
2. Add pepper to your pork.

3. Use a large skillet and cook both sides of your pork in it over medium heat with high-quality extra virgin olive oil until golden brown.

4. Check by a knife to see if the inside pork cooked or not. Remove the pork pieces from the skillet. Add your sauce to the pan and let it cooked for three more minutes.

5. Poach your apple in for 15 minutes in boiling water.

6. Bring back pork pieces to the skillet and let it cook for one more minute.

<u>Cooking Tips:</u>

- This dish can be served with steamed brown rice.

Nutrition Facts

Servings: 4

Amount per serving

Calories	375
	% Daily Value*
Total Fat 15.2g	19%
Saturated Fat 4g	20%
Cholesterol 132mg	44%
Sodium 533mg	23%
Total Carbohydrate 7.4g	3%
Dietary Fiber 0.7g	2%
Total Sugars 5.5g	
Protein 51.3g	
Vitamin D 0mcg	0%
Calcium 7mg	1%
Iron 2mg	10%
Potassium 68mg	1%

BALSAMIC-PEACH PORK

Balsamic-Peach Pork is a great and easy-to-cook meal with few ingredients. A fantastic combination of peach and honey gives the dish a lovely sweet taste.

- Prep Time: 10 minutes
- Cook Time: 20 minutes
- Total Time: 30 minutes
- Serving: 4

<u>Ingredients</u>

- 2 boneless pork tenderloins
- 2 sliced peeled peaches
- 1 tablespoon honey or maple syrup
- 2 tablespoons extra virgin olive oil
- 1 tablespoon fresh chopped oregano or thyme leaves
- Black pepper to taste
- ½ cup fresh basil (optional)

<u>Instructions</u>

1. Mix honey (or maple syrup), oregano, or thyme leaves in a bowl.
2. Add pepper to your pork.
3. Use a large skillet and cook both sides of your pork in it over medium heat with high-quality extra virgin olive oil until golden brown.
4. Check by knife if inside pork cooked well. Remove the pork pieces from the skillet. Add your sauce to the pan and let it cooked for three more minutes.
5. Cook your peeled-off peaches in the same skillet for five minutes. If your sauce gets dry, add water a little bit.
6. Bring back pork pieces to the skillet and let it cook for two more minutes.
7. Garnish with fresh basil if you want. Enjoy!

<u>Cooking Tips:</u>

- This dish can be served well with steamed brown rice.

<u>Diet-related Tips:</u>

- If you cannot tolerate honey, remove honey from your recipe or use one tablespoon of stevia instead.

Nutrition Facts

Servings: 4

Amount per serving

Calories   **266**

	% Daily Value*
Total Fat 15.6g	20%
Saturated Fat 1.5g	8%
Cholesterol 31mg	10%
Sodium 476mg	21%
Total Carbohydrate 14.6g	5%
Dietary Fiber 1.7g	6%
Total Sugars 11.5g	
Protein 18.7g	
Vitamin D 1mcg	6%
Calcium 585mg	45%
Iron 2mg	11%
Potassium 365mg	8%

HONEY-TURMERIC PORK

If you are looking for a healthy dish, you are reading the right recipe. A short cooking-time Honey-Turmeric Pork is an excellent choice for people with rheumatoid arthritis who wants to have a rich main course with pork.

- Prep Time: 15 minutes
- Cook Time: 15 minutes
- Total Time: 30 minutes
- Serving: 4

<u>Ingredients</u>

- 1¼ pounds chopped boneless, fat-removed pork tenderloin
- ½ cup plain yogurt or plain lactose-free yogurt
- ¼ cup honey or maple syrup
- 2 tablespoons extra virgin olive oil
- 3 small carrots
- 1½ teaspoons turmeric powder
- 3 tablespoons fresh lemon juice

- Black pepper to taste
- 3 small beets, sliced thin (optional)

<u>Instructions</u>

1. Mix plain yogurt, honey (or maple syrup), turmeric, and lemon juice in a bowl.
2. Pour pepper on your pork.
3. Use a large skillet and cook both sides of your pork in it over medium heat with high-quality extra virgin olive oil until golden brown.
4. Check by knife if inside pork cooked well. Remove the pork pieces from the skillet. Add your sauce to the pan and let it cooked for three more minutes.
5. Cook your peeled-off beets (optional) and carrots in a small skillet for 10 minutes as sides.
6. Bring back pork pieces to the skillet and let it cook for two more minutes. Enjoy it with carrot and beet sides!

<u>Cooking Tips:</u>

- This dish can be served well with steamed brown rice or brown noodles.
- If you are lactose-intolerant, use lactose-free plain yogurt or remove yogurt from the recipe.

<u>Diet-related Tips:</u>

- If you cannot tolerate honey, remove honey from your recipe or use one tablespoon of stevia instead.

Nutrition Facts

Servings: 4

Amount per serving

Calories	624
	% Daily Value*
Total Fat 18.7g	24%
Saturated Fat 5.2g	26%
Cholesterol 229mg	76%
Sodium 235mg	10%
Total Carbohydrate 26.4g	10%
Dietary Fiber 1.9g	7%
Total Sugars 22.2g	
Protein 84.1g	
Vitamin D 0mcg	0%
Calcium 98mg	8%
Iron 5mg	28%
Potassium 1633mg	35%

GRILLED LEAN OSTRICH MEAT KEBAB

People with rheumatoid arthritis have to significantly reduce red meat in their diet as typically, red meat meals can cause flare-ups. People with rheumatoid arthritis might use extra-lean ostrich meat with no fats in moderation. Ostrich meat tastes very similar to lean beef, but it has less fat, cholesterol. It is high in calcium, iron, and protein. Ask your doctor or nutritionist about the ostrich meat and consume it only if you are allowed.

- Prep Time: 10 minutes
- Marinate Time: 60 minutes
- Cook Time: 20 minutes
- Total Time: 90 minutes
- Serving: 4

<u>Ingredients</u>

- 2 lbs extra lean ostrich meat
- ½ cup plain yogurt or plain lactose-free yogurt
- 1 small kiwi
- 1 onion (thinly sliced)
- 1 tablespoon extra virgin olive oil

- 4 tablespoons fresh lemon juice
- Black pepper to taste

<u>Instructions</u>

1. Cut extra lean ostrich meat into small 1-inch (~2.54cm) cubes.
2. Ina large bowl, marinate your meat with plain yogurt, onion, kiwi, lemon juice, olive oil, and pepper.
3. Cover the top bowl, fridge it and Let it marinate for 1 hour.
4. Skewer your kebab cubes or just grill both sides like a steak. Ten minutes grill would suffice for medium kebabs, and 20 minutes grill would suffice for well-done kebabs.

<u>Cooking Tips:</u>

- You do not necessarily need to cut your meat into cubes. You can flatten them by mallet and make a fantastic steak.
- Kiwi melts your kebab and makes it very juicy.
- If you are lactose-intolerant, use lactose-free plain yogurt or remove yogurt from the recipe.
- If you cannot tolerate ostrich meat, you can use chicken instead of ostrich meat in this recipe.

<u>Diet-related Tips:</u>

- Do not use red meat during flares.
- Try your tolerance regarding ostrich meat in remission periods. Use this recipe only when you are sure that you can tolerate ostrich meat.

HUNGARIAN GOULASH

Goulash is a great traditional stew full of healthy ingredients. People with rheumatoid arthritis need to add chicken, or vegetable broth meals in their diet.

- Prep Time: 30 minutes
- Cook Time: 90 minutes
- Total Time: 120 minutes
- Serving: 6

<u>Ingredients</u>

- 1½ lbs extra lean ostrich meat trimmed into 1 inch (~2.54 cm) cubes
- 2 cups chicken broth or tap water
- 2 tablespoons extra virgin olive oil
- 2 tablespoons lemon juice
- ½ tablespoon turmeric
- ¼ teaspoon pepper
- 1 cup carrots
- 1 cup red/purple potatoes, cut into 1 inch (~2.54cm) cubes
- 1 tablespoon tomato paste (optional)

Instructions

1. One a large pan or a pot, heat olive oil, turmeric, tomato paste (optional), and pepper over medium heat.
2. Add your extra lean ostrich meat and stir for 5 minutes.
3. Add water or chicken broth slowly to your pot. Then, cover and let it cook for 50 minutes over low heat until tender.
4. Add potatoes and let it cook for 20 more minutes. Add lemon juice. Then, add the carrots and cook the stew for 15 more minutes. Enjoy!

<u>Cooking Tips:</u>

- This dish can be served well with steamed brown rice.
- Anytime the stew gets very thick, add more water into it.

<u>Diet-related Tips:</u>

- Use tomato paste only if you can tolerate it.
- Use red/purple potato only if you can tolerate it.
- Ask your doctor or nutritionist about the ostrich meat and consume it only if you are allowed.

TOMATO FREE SPAGHETTI BOLOGNESE

Some rheumatoid arthritis patients cannot tolerate tomatoes and tomato pastes well, which can negatively affect their regular cooking habits using tomatoes inside meals. Let us try a great Spaghetti Bolognese tomato-free! Yes, you read correctly! Enjoy a tomato-free Italian dish now!

- Prep Time: 15 minutes
- Cook Time: 25 minutes
- Total Time: 40 minutes
- Serving: 4

<u>Ingredients</u>

- 1 lb (~500 s) ground extra lean pork or ostrich meat
- 0.65 lb (~300 g) brown rice spaghetti or gluten-free spaghetti
- 1 cup organic unsalted chicken stock
- 1 tablespoon extra virgin olive oil
- 1 tablespoon low sodium soy sauce
- 2 tablespoons maple syrup
- 1 teaspoon dried oregano or oregano powder
- ½ teaspoon dried thyme

- 1 teaspoon dried basil
- ½ tablespoon turmeric
- ¼ teaspoon pepper

<u>Instructions</u>

1. Golden both sides of your extra lean ground ostrich meat in a large pan with extra virgin olive oil over high heat.
2. Add soy sauce, honey (or maple syrup), pepper, turmeric, and chicken stock to your ground meat. Let it thicken and have it cooked for one more minute.
3. At the same time, prepare your spaghetti according to its package recipe with a little bit of olive oil.
4. Take your spaghetti out of boiling water and put it in your sauce.
5. Season it with dried basil.

<u>Cooking Tips:</u>

- If your sauce thickened more than desired, add some tap water or spaghetti boiling water.

<u>Diet-related Tips:</u>

- Ask your doctor or nutritionist about the ostrich meat and consume it only if you are allowed.

GRILLED HONEY SALMON

Try a yummy grilled honey salmon dish.

- Prep Time: 5 minutes
- Cook Time: 25 minutes
- Total Time: 30 minutes
- Serving: 4

Ingredients:

- 2 lbs (~1 kg) salmon fillets
- ¼ cup honey or maple syrup
- 1 tablespoon extra virgin olive oil
- 1 teaspoon turmeric powder
- 1 tablespoon fresh thyme leaves
- Black pepper, to taste

Directions:

1. Choose a medium bowl and whisk honey (or maple syrup), turmeric, thyme leaves, extra virgin olive oil, and pepper together.
2. Preheat your oven to 375 °F.
3. Pour your sauce over the salmon.

4. Put your salmon in the oven and let it cook for 20 minutes (until inside cooks well).
5. Enjoy!

<u>Cooking Tips:</u>

- If your salmon is thicker, you have to increase the cooking time until inside cooks well.
- You can cover your salmon with foil for having a juicy texture.

<u>Diet-related Tips:</u>

- If you cannot tolerate honey, try maple syrup, agave syrup or a teaspoon of stevia.

Nutrition Facts

Servings: 4

Amount per serving

Calories	398
	% Daily Value*
Total Fat 17.6g	23%
Saturated Fat 2.5g	13%
Cholesterol 100mg	33%
Sodium 101mg	4%
Total Carbohydrate 18.3g	7%
Dietary Fiber 0.4g	2%
Total Sugars 17.4g	
Protein 44.2g	
Vitamin D 0mcg	0%
Calcium 95mg	7%
Iron 3mg	15%
Potassium 902mg	19%

Oven-based Salmon and Red Potato

A great mix of salmon and oven-baked potatoes give you a joyful lunch or dinner meal!

- Prep Time: 5 minutes
- Cook Time: 25 minutes
- Total Time: 30 minutes
- Serving: 4

<u>Ingredients</u>

- 4 salmon filets, about 6 ounces each
- 2 medium red/purple potatoes, sliced into very thin chips
- 3 tablespoons extra-virgin olive oil, divided
- 2 oranges
- 2 lemons
- Pepper, to taste

<u>Instructions</u>

1. Choose a small bowl and whisk orange juice, lemon juice, 1 tablespoon of extra virgin olive oil, and pepper all together to have a juicy sauce.
2. Marinate your salmon with the sauce.
3. Slice potatoes very thin. Drizzle potatoes with two tablespoons of extra virgin olive oil.
4. Preheat your oven to 375 °F.
5. Choose a long foil sheet, put potatoes first, and fill the top with your salmon. Close your foil and let the salmon cook for about 25 minutes until inside cooks well.
6. Enjoy!

<u>Cooking Tips:</u>

- If your salmon is very thick, you have to increase the cooking time until inside cooks well.
- Check both salmon and your potato to be cooked. If required, return your salmon and potato to the over for five more minutes until perfection.

<u>Diet-related Tips:</u>

- If you cannot tolerate orange juice, remove it from the recipe.
- Remove red/purple potato from the recipe if you cannot tolerate it.

Nutrition Facts

Servings: 4

Amount per serving

Calories	**443**
	% Daily Value*
Total Fat 21.8g	28%
Saturated Fat 3.1g	16%
Cholesterol 78mg	26%
Sodium 84mg	4%
Total Carbohydrate 28.4g	10%
Dietary Fiber 4.9g	18%
Total Sugars 10g	
Protein 37.4g	
Vitamin D 0mcg	0%
Calcium 117mg	9%
Iron 2mg	11%
Potassium 1248mg	27%

LEMON STEAMED HALIBUT WITH BROWN RICE

A great dish with healthy ingredients for people with rheumatoid arthritis. You can substitute halibut with any types of fish you would like to have.

- Prep Time: 10 minutes
- Cook Time: 30 minutes
- Total Time: 40 minutes
- Serving: 6

<u>Ingredients</u>

- 6 skinless and boneless halibut fillets, about 6 ounces each
- 2 cups steamed brown rice
- 1 tablespoon extra virgin olive oil
- 1 lemon, sliced very thin
- 4 tablespoons lemon juice
- 1 teaspoon ginger powder

- Pepper to taste
- Lemon wedges to garnish

Instructions

1. Choose a small bowl and whisk lemon juice, ginger powder, extra virgin olive oil, and pepper all together to have a juicy sauce.
2. Marinate your halibut with the sauce.
3. Preheat your oven to 375 °F.
4. Choose a long foil sheet, put halibut in your foil sheet, and close it. Let it cook for about 25 minutes until inside cooks well.
5. Open the foil sheet, put thin lemon slices on top of your halibut for 5 minutes, and close the foil sheet again.
6. Steam your brown rice. Open your foil sheet and put halibut on top of the rice.
7. Garnish with lemon wedges. Enjoy!

Cooking Tips:

- If your halibut is very thick, you have to increase the cooking time until inside cooks well.

Nutrition Facts

Servings: 6

Amount per serving

Calories	568
	% Daily Value*
Total Fat 9.5g	12%
Saturated Fat 1.4g	7%
Cholesterol 93mg	31%
Sodium 161mg	7%
Total Carbohydrate 50.2g	18%
Dietary Fiber 1.3g	4%
Total Sugars 0.3g	
Protein 65g	
Vitamin D 0mcg	0%
Calcium 33mg	3%
Iron 16mg	87%
Potassium 1396mg	30%

THUNFISCH PIZZA

Thunfisch Pizza is an excellent German-based pizza with Tuna. The classic recipe has been modified to be tolerated by most people with rheumatoid arthritis.

- Prep Time: 5 minutes
- Cook Time: 15 minutes
- Total Time: 20 minutes
- Serving: 4

<u>Ingredients</u>

- 2 medium-size gluten-free pizza crusts
- 1 cup shredded dairy-free cheese pizza
- Two 6.5 oz tuna can on extra virgin olive oil or water
- 2 tablespoons organic mayonnaise
- 2 teaspoons dried ground oregano

<u>Instructions</u>

1. Place your gluten-free pizza crusts on a non-stick pizza pan or bake sheet.
2. Spread your organic mayo on your crust.
3. Gently put tuna on your pizza crust.
4. Sprinkle with dairy-free cheese
5. Let it bake at 400 °F for 10 minutes. Then, broil on the same heat for five more minutes until cheese melted.

<u>Diet-related Tips:</u>

- Use mayonnaise only if you can tolerate it. If you cannot tolerate, you can make a béchamel sauce (explain before in Fettuccine Alfredo recipe) instead.

Nutrition Facts

Servings: 4

Amount per serving

Calories	297
	% Daily Value*
Total Fat 13g	17%
Saturated Fat 2.9g	14%
Cholesterol 33mg	11%
Sodium 333mg	14%
Total Carbohydrate 17g	6%
Dietary Fiber 0.8g	3%
Total Sugars 1.5g	
Protein 26.8g	
Vitamin D 0mcg	0%
Calcium 21mg	2%
Iron 1mg	5%
Potassium 310mg	7%

Avocado Tuna Pita

A very fast sandwich you can prepare at home for your lunch or dinner. You can even have a smaller portion of avocado tuna as a breakfast or as a snack at work.

- Prep Time: 10 minutes
- Cook Time: 0 minutes
- Total Time: 10 minutes
- Serving: 4

Ingredients

- 2 avocados
- 2 tablespoons organic low-sodium mayonnaise
- 1 teaspoon cumin powder
- 1 can of tuna in olive oil or water
- ¼ cup apple, chopped and peeled off
- 4 Pita bread or gluten-free pita/bread
- Pepper to taste (optional)

Instructions

1. Choose a small bowl. Mix tuna with smashed avocado with mayo, cumin powder, peeled off apple (cut into small pieces), and pepper (optional).
2. Open each of your pita bread from the corner and spoon the mix inside.
3. Roll the pita. Enjoy!

<u>Cooking Tips:</u>

- You can make this sandwich without mayonnaise sauce, as well.

Nutrition Facts

Servings: 4

Amount per serving

Calories	491
	% Daily Value*
Total Fat 26.5g	34%
Saturated Fat 5.3g	27%
Cholesterol 16mg	5%
Sodium 442mg	19%
Total Carbohydrate 46g	17%
Dietary Fiber 8.5g	30%
Total Sugars 3.2g	
Protein 19.4g	
Vitamin D 0mcg	0%
Calcium 71mg	5%
Iron 3mg	16%
Potassium 733mg	16%

TROUT WITH ORANGE

Great classic seafood that typically serves with steamed brown rice. It is recommended to make this dish with bitter or blood oranges.

- Prep Time: 20 minutes
- Cook Time: 30 minutes
- Total Time: 50 minutes
- Serving: 6

<u>Ingredients</u>

- Large fresh trout, 1.5 lbs each
- 3 oranges
- 1 tablespoon lemon juice
- 1 tablespoon extra virgin olive oil
- ½ teaspoon turmeric powder
- Pepper to taste

<u>Instructions</u>

1. Choose a medium bowl and whisk lemon juice, orange juice, turmeric powder, extra virgin olive oil, and pepper all together to have a juicy sauce.
2. Marinate your trout with the sauce. For better taste, you may need to let it rest at room temperature for 30 minutes.
3. Preheat your oven to 375 °F.
4. Choose a long foil sheet, put trout in your foil sheet and close it. Let it cook for about 25 minutes until inside cooks well.
5. Enjoy!

<u>Cooking Tips:</u>

- Check your trout until inside cooked well. You may need more minutes for perfection.
- You can substitute orange with mango or lemon juice if you like to try other great flavors.

Nutrition Facts

Servings: 4

Amount per serving

Calories   **391**

	% Daily Value*
Total Fat 16.9g	22%
Saturated Fat 2.8g	14%
Cholesterol 115mg	38%
Sodium 105mg	5%
Total Carbohydrate 16.5g	6%
Dietary Fiber 3.4g	12%
Total Sugars 13g	
Protein 42.6g	
Vitamin D 0mcg	0%
Calcium 141mg	11%
Iron 3mg	18%
Potassium 980mg	21%

CHICKEN AND SHRIMP TERIYAKI

A lovely Edo-style mix of chicken and shrimp with healthy ingredients for people with rheumatoid arthritis.

- Prep Time: 5 minutes
- Cook Time: 20 minutes
- Total Time: 25 minutes
- Serving: 4

<u>Ingredients</u>

- 2 lbs (~1 kg) organic chicken breast, chopped in cubes
- 20 shrimps, peeled and deveined
- 1 tablespoon ginger powder, divided
- 2 tablespoons extra virgin olive oil
- ½ teaspoon turmeric
- ⅓ cup gluten-free and sodium-reduced soy sauce
- ⅓ cup of cold water
- 3 teaspoons arrowroot powder
- ¼ cup honey, or maple syrup
- Pepper to taste

<u>Instructions</u>

1. In a medium bowl, whisk ginger powder, one tablespoon of olive oil, soy sauce, arrowroot powder, honey (or maple syrup), water, and pepper to make a juicy teriyaki sauce.
2. Let Teriyaki sauce rest in the fridge for 5 minutes.
3. In a large pan, add one tablespoon of olive oil and cook chicken over medium heat until golden brown both sides.
4. Add your sauce and shrimp to the pan. Stir and mix for 5 minutes until thickened.
5. Enjoy!

<u>Cooking Tips:</u>

- You can serve this dish with steamed brown rice.

<u>Diet-related Tips:</u>

- Use maple syrup or stevia (1 teaspoon) if you cannot tolerate honey.

Nutrition Facts

Servings: 4

Amount per serving

Calories	553
	% Daily Value*
Total Fat 15.1g	19%
Saturated Fat 1.7g	9%
Cholesterol 423mg	141%
Sodium 1639mg	71%
Total Carbohydrate 20g	7%
Dietary Fiber 0.4g	1%
Total Sugars 12.1g	
Protein 79.6g	
Vitamin D 0mcg	1%
Calcium 151mg	12%
Iron 2mg	12%
Potassium 1175mg	25%

Lemon Shrimp with Brown Rice

Lemon Shrimp with steamed brown rice is very easy to make and a healthy dish you can have in your weekly diet.

- Prep Time: 5 minutes
- Cook Time: 20 minutes
- Total Time: 25 minutes
- Serving: 4

Ingredients

- 20 shrimps, peeled and deveined
- 2 tablespoons extra virgin olive oil, divided
- ½ teaspoon turmeric powder
- 4 tablespoons lemon juice
- 3 cups of brown rice
- 1 teaspoon pepper

Instructions

1. In a small bowl, whisk lemon juice, one tablespoon of olive oil, turmeric powder, and pepper to make a sauce.
2. Cook your rice according to its package instructions.
3. Add one tablespoon of high-quality extra virgin olive oil in a pan and cook shrimp over medium heat for 5-7 minutes.
4. Add your sauce into the pan. Stir and mix well for 5 minutes.
5. Enjoy!

Cooking Tips:

- You can serve the lemon shrimp with brown noodles instead of brown rice.

Nutrition Facts

Servings: 4

Amount per serving

Calories	729
	% Daily Value*
Total Fat 10.3g	13%
Saturated Fat 2.1g	10%
Cholesterol 278mg	93%
Sodium 332mg	14%
Total Carbohydrate 113.8g	41%
Dietary Fiber 2.1g	7%
Total Sugars 0.5g	
Protein 40.2g	
Vitamin D 0mcg	0%
Calcium 162mg	12%
Iron 7mg	37%
Potassium 416mg	9%

Honey Prawn Linguine

Are you looking for an Italian seafood linguine recipe for people with rheumatoid arthritis? You have to try this delicious main course.

- Prep Time: 5 minutes
- Cook Time: 20 minutes
- Total Time: 25 minutes
- Serving: 4

Ingredients:

- 1 lb (~500 gr) prawns, peeled and deveined
- 1 lb (~500 gr) cooked gluten-free linguine or any other types of brown rice or quinoa pasta
- 2 tablespoons extra virgin olive oil, divided
- 4 tablespoons honey or maple syrup
- ½ cup carrot
- ½ cup of water
- Black pepper to taste
- ¼ cup green onion (only if tolerated)

Instructions

1. Whisk honey (or maple syrup), one tablespoon of olive oil, carrot, green onion, and pepper in a proper bowl to make a sauce.
2. Cook your linguini according to its package instructions.
3. Add one tablespoon of high-quality extra virgin olive oil in a medium-size pan and cook prawns over medium heat for 5-7 minutes.
4. Add your sauce into the pan. Stir and mix well for 5 minutes until sauce gets thick.
5. Add pasta to your sauce and mix all well. Enjoy!

<u>Diet-related Tips:</u>

- You can use maple syrup, agave syrup, or a teaspoon of stevia if you cannot tolerate honey.

Nutrition Facts

Servings: 4

Amount per serving

Calories	592
	% Daily Value*
Total Fat 11.5g	15%
Saturated Fat 2g	10%
Cholesterol 322mg	107%
Sodium 317mg	14%
Total Carbohydrate 82.7g	30%
Dietary Fiber 0.5g	2%
Total Sugars 18g	
Protein 38.9g	
Vitamin D 0mcg	0%
Calcium 128mg	10%
Iron 4mg	24%
Potassium 461mg	10%

DESSERTS

PEAR CAKE SUNDAES

A delicious dessert with pear, cinnamon, and ice cream. Substantially modified to be consumed by people with rheumatoid arthritis.

- Prep Time: 15 minutes
- Total Time: 15 minutes
- Serving: 4

<u>Ingredients</u>

- 2 tablespoons extra virgin olive oil
- 1 tablespoon honey
- 1 cup pear, chopped
- 1-pint dairy-free vanilla ice cream or sorbet
- 1½ cup vanilla loaf pound cake
- 1 tablespoon maple syrup
- ¼ teaspoon cinnamon powder

<u>Instructions</u>

- In a medium skillet, heat extra virgin olive oil over medium heat. Add cinnamon, and honey. Stir well until brown with a soft texture.
- Add pear and let it cook for two-three more minutes. Remove from heat.
- Preheat oven to 375 °F. Bake your cake for about 8-10 minutes until toasted.
- Crumble vanilla loaf pound cake and place it on top of ice cream scoops (or sorbets). Pour maple syrup on top.
- Add pear sauce. Serve and enjoy!

<u>Cooking Tips:</u>

- You can mix the pear sauce with any cold plain or vanilla yogurt instead of ice cream.

<u>Diet-related Tips:</u>

- Remember to always avoid refined sugars. Instead, you can use honey. If you cannot tolerate honey well, you can use maple syrup or stevia.

Nutrition Facts
Servings: 4

Amount per serving

Calories	213
	% Daily Value*
Total Fat 10.8g	14%
Saturated Fat 2.6g	13%
Cholesterol 12mg	4%
Sodium 54mg	2%
Total Carbohydrate 29g	11%
Dietary Fiber 0.7g	3%
Total Sugars 23.5g	
Protein 1.4g	
Vitamin D 0mcg	0%
Calcium 41mg	3%
Iron 1mg	3%
Potassium 78mg	2%

APPLE-GINGER SUNDAES

This summer sundae is based on a great combination of apple, ginger, and ice cream.

- Prep Time: 20 minutes
- Total Time: 20 minutes
- Serving: 4

Ingredients

- 2 apples, peeled and sliced
- 2 tablespoons extra virgin olive oil
- 2 tablespoons honey
- 6 tablespoons organic no added sugar, apple juice
- ½ teaspoon cornstarch
- 2 cup dairy-free vanilla ice cream or sorbet
- ¼ teaspoon freshly grated ginger

Instructions

- In a large skillet, heat extra virgin olive oil over medium heat. Add apple and ginger and cook for three minutes until tender. Add honey and stir well for 1-2 minutes.
- In a bowl, mix cornstarch and apple juice and pour the mix into the skillet. Cook all mix until thickened.
- Cool for 2-4 minutes.
- Scoop your ice cream or sorbet in a proper dessert plate. Pour your apple ginger mix on top.
- Serve and enjoy!

<u>Cooking Tips:</u>

- You can mix the apple ginger sauce with any cold plain or vanilla yogurt instead of ice cream.

<u>Diet-related Tips:</u>

- Remember to always avoid refined sugars. Instead, you can use honey. If you cannot tolerate honey well, you can use maple syrup or stevia.
- If you cannot tolerate cornstarch well, use almond flour or rice flour.

Nutrition Facts

Servings: 4

Amount per serving

Calories	**212**
	% Daily Value*
Total Fat 10.7g	14%
Saturated Fat 3.3g	16%
Cholesterol 10mg	3%
Sodium 20mg	1%
Total Carbohydrate 29.7g	11%
Dietary Fiber 2.7g	10%
Total Sugars 25.2g	
Protein 1.3g	
Vitamin D 0mcg	0%
Calcium 46mg	4%
Iron 1mg	3%
Potassium 151mg	3%

Banana Lemon Trifle

If you want to try a different delicious dessert, you have to make Banana Lemon Trifle.

- Prep Time: 10 minutes
- Total Time: 20 minutes
- Serving: 6

Ingredients

- 4 packs instant vanilla pudding or gluten-free vanilla pudding
- 3 packs gluten-free shortbread cookies
- ½ cup almond milk
- 3 bananas, sliced
- 1 tablespoon lemon juice
- Lemon zest
- 4-5 fresh mint leaves

Instructions

- In a large bowl, prepare vanilla pudding according to package instructions. Then mix pudding with lemon juice, lemon zest, and almond milk.
- Top the bowl with shredded shortbread cookies and sliced banana. Garnish with mint leaves.

Cooking Tips:

- You can top the bowl with cinnamon powder as well.

Nutrition Facts

Servings: 6

Amount per serving

Calories 481

% Daily Value*

Total Fat 11.2g	14%
Saturated Fat 6.4g	32%
Cholesterol 28mg	9%
Sodium 1033mg	45%
Total Carbohydrate 94.1g	34%
Dietary Fiber 2.6g	9%
Total Sugars 74.3g	
Protein 2.4g	
Vitamin D 0mcg	0%
Calcium 21mg	2%
Iron 1mg	4%
Potassium 253mg	5%

Warm Apple Crumble

Warm apple crumble is a quick dessert to make for yourself and your family.

- Prep Time: 15 minutes
- Cook Time: 15 minutes
- Total Time: 30 minutes
- Serving: 4

<u>Ingredients</u>

- 2.5 cups apple, peeled and sliced
- 1 teaspoon vanilla extract
- 2 tablespoons honey
- 1 teaspoon cinnamon powder, divided
- 2 tablespoons extra virgin olive oil
- Dairy-free vanilla ice cream or sorbet (optional)

<u>Instructions</u>

1. In a medium bowl, mix apple, with vanilla, sugar or honey, and half-teaspoon cinnamon powder.
2. Preheat oven to 350 °F.
3. Choose a proper baking dish. Place the mix in it.

4. Bake apples until slightly get golden (about 12-15 minutes).
5. Serve the apple crumble warm (with or without vanilla ice cream or sorbet). Enjoy!

<u>Cooking Tips:</u>

- Your cooking time highly depends on how thin you sliced apples. Keep your eyes on apples to avoid overcooking.

<u>Diet-related Tips:</u>

- Remember to always avoid refined sugars. Instead, you can use honey. If you cannot tolerate honey well, you can use maple syrup or stevia.

Nutrition Facts

Servings: 4

Amount per serving

Calories	177
	% Daily Value*
Total Fat 8.9g	11%
Saturated Fat 2.5g	12%
Cholesterol 0mg	0%
Sodium 2mg	0%
Total Carbohydrate 26.6g	10%
Dietary Fiber 4.1g	15%
Total Sugars 21g	
Protein 0.6g	
Vitamin D 0mcg	0%
Calcium 7mg	1%
Iron 1mg	8%
Potassium 171mg	4%

Apple Quesadillas

If you can tolerate tortilla, then this dessert is an excellent option for you to make. It perfectly comes with ice cream on top.

- Prep Time: 10 minutes
- Cook Time: 10 minutes

- Total Time: 20 minutes
- Serving: 4-6

<u>Ingredients</u>

- 4 pieces of tortillas
- 1 tablespoon extra virgin olive oil
- 2 large apples, peeled, cored and skin removed
- 2 tablespoons honey
- 4 tablespoons dairy-free ice cream or sorbet

<u>Instructions</u>

1. Preheat oven to 375 °F.
2. Place your tortillas on a proper baking sheet. Sprinkle extra virgin olive oil, and top with honey, and thinly sliced apples on half of each tortilla.
3. Wrap tortilla by folding the other half towards the half with mixture.
4. Bake quesadillas for about 7-10 minutes until golden.
5. Scoop ice cream or sorbet and top it with your apple mix. Enjoy!

<u>Cooking Tips:</u>

- You can use poached apple or warmed canned apple instead. Dice them and top with other ingredients. Cook for 5 minutes.

<u>Diet-related Tips:</u>

- Remember to always avoid refined sugars. Instead, you can use honey. If you cannot tolerate honey well, you can use maple syrup or stevia.

GLUTEN-FREE APPLE PIE

This homemade gluten-free apple pie made with almond flour can satisfy you and your gut!

- Prep Time: 30 minutes
- Cook Time: 55 minutes
- Total Time: 85 minutes
- Serving: 6

Ingredients

- 1¾ cups almond flour, grounded
- ¼ cup tapioca flour+2 tablespoons tapioca flour
- 6 tablespoons extra virgin olive oil
- ½ large egg whisked
- 1 cup rolled oats
- 1 cup + ½ tablespoon honey
- 1 teaspoon cinnamon powder
- ½ teaspoon ground ginger
- 4 apples, peeled, cored and sliced
- 1 tablespoon lemon juice
- 1 tablespoon vanilla extract

Instructions

1. In a large bowl, mix almond and tapioca flour rolled oats and olive oil.
2. In a bowl, whisk egg a bit and adds ½ of an egg into the dough. Mix well to form a soft-ball. If the texture is not good, add 1 or 2 teaspoons of the whisked egg to the dough.
3. Put your dough on a parchment paper. Fridge the dough for an hour (Recommended keeping it in a fridge overnight).
4. Remove from the fridge. With a rolling pin, make a 10-12 inch disk. Then, gently move your dough disk to the pie plate. Return into its shape again if any part falls apart or breaks.
5. Crimp the edges with your fingertips. Make small holes in all parts of your dough.
6. In a large bowl, mix thinly sliced apples with lemon juice, vanilla extract, sugar or honey, and ginger.
7. Cover your crust with the mix altogether.
8. Preheat oven to 400 °F.
9. Cover crust edges with a pie shield to avoid burning fast.
10. Bake for 15-20 minutes. Reduce heat to 350°F and let it bake for 40 minutes.
11. Remove from the oven. Cool down. Slice it and serve.

Cooking Tips:

- Cover the pie with aluminum foil if you see the toppings are getting brown so fast.

Diet-related Tips:

- If you cannot tolerate honey well, you can use maple syrup or stevia.

Nutrition Facts

Servings: 6

Amount per serving	
Calories	**380**
	% Daily Value*
Total Fat 23.4g	30%
Saturated Fat 2.8g	14%
Cholesterol 14mg	5%
Sodium 18mg	1%
Total Carbohydrate 40.5g	15%
Dietary Fiber 6.1g	22%
Total Sugars 16.5g	
Protein 5.3g	
Vitamin D 1mcg	6%
Calcium 43mg	3%
Iron 2mg	10%
Potassium 299mg	6%

Pumpkin Pie

Enjoy cooking a traditional pumpkin pie recipe for people with rheumatoid arthritis!

- Prep Time: 15 minutes
- Cook Time: 55 minutes
- Total Time: 70 minutes
- Serving: 4-6

Ingredients

- 2 cups pumpkin, peeled
- 1 ready pie crust, gluten-free (9-inch)
- 2 organic, free-range eggs
- 1.5 cups lactose-free condensed milk
- ½ teaspoon freshly grated ginger
- ½ teaspoon cinnamon powder

Instructions

1. Preheat oven to 400°F.

2. Blend the pumpkin with all other ingredients in a blender or whisk all ingredients in a large bowl.
3. Pour the mix in a ready crust and bake for 15 minutes.
4. Reduce heat to 350 °F and let it bake for 35-40 minutes. You can insert a fork into it. The fork has to come out very clean, showing that it perfectly cooked.
5. Serve and enjoy!

Cooking Tips:

- Cover the pie with aluminum foil if you see the toppings are getting brown so fast.

Diet-related Tips:

- Make sure you can tolerate condensed milk. If you cannot, use almond milk instead.

Nutrition Facts

Servings: 6

Amount per serving

Calories	403
	% Daily Value*
Total Fat 15.3g	20%
Saturated Fat 5.8g	29%
Cholesterol 81mg	27%
Sodium 258mg	11%
Total Carbohydrate 58.9g	21%
Dietary Fiber 2.6g	9%
Total Sugars 45.3g	
Protein 9.7g	
Vitamin D 5mcg	26%
Calcium 251mg	19%
Iron 2mg	11%
Potassium 497mg	11%

Fruit Dessert

A fresh cold fruit mix as a healthy dessert choice for people with rheumatoid arthritis.

- Prep Time: 20 minutes

- Total Time: 20 minutes
- Serving: 4

Ingredients

- 2 cups cantaloupe, cubed
- 2 cups mix pf different berries, cubed
- 1 tablespoon maple syrup
- 3 tablespoons lime juice
- 1 cup papaya, cubed
- 2 cups honeydew melon, cubed

Instructions

1. In a large bowl, mix all ingredients.
2. Serve cold. Enjoy!

Nutrition Facts

Servings: 4

Amount per serving

Calories	132
	% Daily Value*
Total Fat 0.5g	1%
Saturated Fat 0.1g	1%
Cholesterol 0mg	0%
Sodium 33mg	1%
Total Carbohydrate 34g	12%
Dietary Fiber 3.3g	12%
Total Sugars 27.3g	
Protein 1.8g	
Vitamin D 0mcg	0%
Calcium 36mg	3%
Iron 1mg	4%
Potassium 594mg	13%

Avocado Pear Popsicle

Homemade popsicles are great desserts for people with rheumatoid arthritis. It is very easy to make popsicles at home. You need to try this recipe as an example:

- Prep Time: 10 minutes
- Freeze Time: 90 minutes

- Total Time: 100 minutes
- Serving: 4

Ingredients

- 2 avocados, peeled
- 2 pears, peeled and cored

Instructions

1. Blend well pears and avocados in a blender or food processor.
2. Fill up your Popsicle cups. Insert popsicle sticks and freeze.
3. Run the outside of the cup under hot water to remove the popsicles when you want to eat it.

Cooking Tips:

- You can change the fruit(s) in your popsicle as you wish, but make sure you can tolerate those fruits and always peel them off. Berries and dark grapes are great options for making popsicles.

Diet-related Tips:

- Peel and poach fruits such as apple, pear, or peach if you want to make a Popsicle from them.

LEMON SORBET

Try a Paleo-kind refreshing sorbet with great combinations of lemon juice and honey.

- Prep Time: 10 minutes
- Make Time: 120 minutes
- Total Time: 130 minutes
- Serving: 4

Ingredients

- 1 cup fresh lemon juice
- 2 tablespoons lemon zest
- 2 cups of water
- ½ cup honey or maple syrup
- ¼ teaspoon vanilla extract

Instructions

1. In a medium pot, mix your honey (or maple syrup), lemon zest, and water until the honey dissolves and gets warm.
2. Add lemon juice or squeeze a lemon to the pot. Stir a bit.

3. Pour your sorbet mixture into a metal pan or pot or an ice cream maker.
4. Freeze for 2 hours. Scrape the sorbet with a spoon or fork every 15 minutes.
5. Enjoy!

<u>Cooking Tips:</u>

- You can change the fruit(s) in your sorbet as you wish, but make sure you can tolerate those fruits and always peel them off. Some fruits need to be cooked before making the sorbet.

<u>Diet-related Tips:</u>

- Peel and poach fruits such as apple, pear, or peach if you want to make a sorbet from them.

Nutrition Facts

Servings: 4

Amount per serving

Calories	234

% Daily Value*

Total Fat 9.8g	13%
Saturated Fat 6.3g	31%
Cholesterol 33mg	11%
Sodium 24mg	1%
Total Carbohydrate 37.7g	14%
Dietary Fiber 0.5g	2%
Total Sugars 36.3g	
Protein 1.3g	
Vitamin D 0mcg	0%
Calcium 29mg	2%
Iron 0mg	1%
Potassium 136mg	3%

MANGO ICE CREAM

This dairy-free mango ice cream is very easy to make. It is healthy and a tasty dessert choice for people with rheumatoid arthritis.

- Prep Time: 15 minutes

- Cook Time: 30 minutes
- Total Time: 45 minutes
- Serving: 6

Ingredients

- 1¾ cup almond milk
- 2 mangos, peeled
- ¼ cup honey or maple syrup
- ½ teaspoon vanilla extract

Instructions

1. Perfectly chill your almond milk in a fridge before you make this ice cream.
2. Blend milk, mango, maple syrup, and vanilla extract in a blender until perfectly smooth.
3. Pour your sorbet mixture into a metal container, pot, or an ice cream maker. If you use an ice cream maker, it takes about 30 minutes, but if you use a metal container, you may need to freeze it for 90-120 minutes.
4. Serve cold and enjoy it!

Cooking Tips:

- You can change the fruits in your ice cream as you desire, but make sure you can tolerate those fruits and always peel them off. Making ice creams from berries are great people with RA.

White Panna Cotta

A dairy-free, easy to make panna cotta for people with rheumatoid arthritis that comes with a lovely creamy taste of almond milk.

- Prep Time: 10 minutes
- Chill time: 120 minutes
- Total Time: 130 minutes
- Serving: 4

Ingredients

- 1¾ cup almond milk
- ⅓ cup maple syrup or honey
- 2 teaspoons gelatin, grass-fed
- 1 teaspoon vanilla extract

Instructions

1. In a medium pan, heat almond milk and add gelatin. Stir until gelatin powder melts.
2. Add vanilla. Stir and let the mix get warmer for 3-5 minutes over medium heat until gelatin fully dissolved. Be aware that you should not boil the milk.

3. Remove from pan and add maple syrup or honey. Stir well.
4. Fill some small cups with the mixture and fridge it for 3-4 hours.
5. To remove Panna Cotta easily, put small cups in a hot water bowl for 2 minutes. Then, you can flip Panna Cottas on your dessert plates. Enjoy!

Cooking Tips:

- For having a fruity Panna Cotta, you can add poached and peeled fruit cubes in your mixture, as well.
- Alternatively, you can garnish your panna cotta with fruits you can tolerate such as berries.

Nutrition Facts
Servings: 4

Amount per serving

Calories	325
	% Daily Value*
Total Fat 25.1g	32%
Saturated Fat 22.2g	111%
Cholesterol 0mg	0%
Sodium 25mg	1%
Total Carbohydrate 23.6g	9%
Dietary Fiber 2.3g	8%
Total Sugars 19.3g	
Protein 5.4g	
Vitamin D 0mcg	0%
Calcium 36mg	3%
Iron 2mg	12%
Potassium 332mg	7%

COCKTAILS AND SHAKES

BANANA MILKSHAKE

Enjoy tasting a traditional milkshake with banana.

- Prep Time: 5 minutes
- Serving: 1

Ingredients

- 1 banana
- 1 cup unsweetened almond
- ½ teaspoon stevia or two tablespoons honey or maple syrup

Instructions

- Blend all the above ingredients until smooth. Pour into a large glass. Enjoy!

Cooking Tips:

- Use agave syrup if you cannot tolerate maple syrup or honey.

Diet-related Tips:

- Use honey only if you can tolerate it.

Nutrition Facts

Servings: 1

Amount per serving

Calories	145
	% Daily Value*
Total Fat 3.9g	5%
Saturated Fat 0.4g	2%
Cholesterol 0mg	0%
Sodium 181mg	8%
Total Carbohydrate 29g	11%
Dietary Fiber 4.1g	15%
Total Sugars 14.4g	
Protein 2.3g	
Vitamin D .1mcg	7%
Calcium 306mg	24%
Iron 1mg	6%
Potassium 612mg	13%

COOLER DRINK

Enjoy tasting a great drink that makes you really cool!

- Prep Time: 5 minutes
- Serving: 1

<u>Ingredients</u>

- 2 cucumbers, peeled
- 10 mint leaves
- 1 cup lemon juice
- 1 cup of water
- Ice cubes

<u>Instructions</u>

- Blend all ingredients in a blender and then blend until smooth. Pour into a large glass. Enjoy!

<u>Cooking Tips:</u>

- You can add one teaspoon of freshly grated ginger to the drink as well.

Nutrition Facts

Servings: 1

Amount per serving

Calories	193
	% Daily Value*
Total Fat 3.3g	4%
Saturated Fat 2.4g	12%
Cholesterol 0mg	0%
Sodium 91mg	4%
Total Carbohydrate 35.4g	13%
Dietary Fiber 10.8g	39%
Total Sugars 15.2g	
Protein 9.2g	
Vitamin D 0mcg	0%
Calcium 312mg	24%
Iron 14mg	76%
Potassium 1646mg	35%

MANGO-BANANA SMOOTHIE

A great smoothie with mango and banana!

- Prep Time: 5 minutes
- Serving: 1-2

<u>Ingredients</u>

- 1 mango, diced
- 1 banana, diced
- 1 cup almond milk
- ½ teaspoon stevia (or honey or maple syrup)

<u>Instructions</u>

- Blend all ingredients in a blender and then blend until smooth. Pour into a large glass. Enjoy!

<u>Cooking Tips:</u>

- Use agave syrup if you cannot tolerate maple syrup or honey.

<u>Diet-related Tips:</u>

- Use honey only if you can tolerate it.
- If you cannot tolerate mango, use papaya instead.

Nutrition Facts

Servings: 2

Amount per serving

Calories	218
	% Daily Value*
Total Fat 3.4g	4%
Saturated Fat 1.7g	9%
Cholesterol 11mg	4%
Sodium 62mg	3%
Total Carbohydrate 44.7g	16%
Dietary Fiber 4.2g	15%
Total Sugars 30.2g	
Protein 6.3g	
Vitamin D 50mcg	250%
Calcium 171mg	13%
Iron 0mg	2%
Potassium 703mg	15%

GINGER COOL DRINK

A great healthy drink for people with rheumatoid arthritis.

- Prep Time: 5 minutes

- Serving: 1

Ingredients

- 5 tablespoons applesauce
- 1 cup of water
- 1 cup of cooked pear or 1 can of pear compote
- 1 small piece of ginger or 2 teaspoons ginger powder

Instructions

- Blend all ingredients in a blender and then blend until smooth. Pour into a large glass. Enjoy!

Cooking Tips:

- You can add honey (if you can tolerate) or ½ tablespoon of stevia for sweetness.

Nutrition Facts

Servings: 1

Amount per serving

Calories	**138**

% Daily Value*

Total Fat 0.5g	1%
Saturated Fat 0.1g	0%
Cholesterol 0mg	0%
Sodium 5mg	0%
Total Carbohydrate 35.7g	13%
Dietary Fiber 6.4g	23%
Total Sugars 23.5g	
Protein 1g	
Vitamin D 0mcg	0%
Calcium 21mg	2%
Iron 1mg	4%
Potassium 292mg	6%

Avocado Smoothie

A great healthy drink for people with rheumatoid arthritis with healthy fats. If you like, you can add protein powder in the smoothie.

- Prep Time: 5 minutes

- Serving: 1-2

Ingredients

- 1 avocado
- 1 banana
- 1 cup almond milk
- 2 tablespoons maple syrup or 1 teaspoon stevia

Instructions

- Blend all ingredients in a blender and then blend until smooth. Pour into a large glass. Enjoy!

Cooking Tips:

- Use can use honey (if you can tolerate) instead of maple syrup.

Nutrition Facts

Servings: 2

Amount per serving

Calories	375
	% Daily Value*
Total Fat 22.3g	29%
Saturated Fat 5.7g	29%
Cholesterol 10mg	3%
Sodium 71mg	3%
Total Carbohydrate 42g	15%
Dietary Fiber 8.3g	30%
Total Sugars 25.6g	
Protein 6.6g	
Vitamin D 0mcg	0%
Calcium 176mg	14%
Iron 1mg	6%
Potassium 739mg	16%

BANANA-CINNAMON SMOOTHIE

A classical thick smoothie to enjoy!

- Prep Time: 5 minutes
- Serving: 1

Ingredients

- 1 banana
- 1 cup vanilla yogurt or lactose-free yogurt
- 2 teaspoons maple syrup or ½ teaspoon stevia
- 1 teaspoon cinnamon
- ⅓ cup of ice

Instructions

- Blend all ingredients in a blender and then blend until smooth. Pour into a large glass. Enjoy!

Cooking Tips:

- Use can use honey (if you can tolerate) instead of maple syrup.
- Plain yogurt can also be used instead of vanilla yogurt.

Nutrition Facts

Servings: 1

Amount per serving

Calories	320
	% Daily Value*
Total Fat 3.5g	4%
Saturated Fat 2.6g	13%
Cholesterol 15mg	5%
Sodium 174mg	8%
Total Carbohydrate 55g	20%
Dietary Fiber 4.3g	15%
Total Sugars 39.7g	
Protein 15.3g	
Vitamin D 0mcg	0%
Calcium 486mg	37%
Iron 1mg	5%
Potassium 1033mg	22%

PEACH-MANGO-BERRIES SMOOTHIE

A fabulous smoothie with three different fruits to enjoy!

- Prep Time: 5 minutes
- Serving: 1-2

Ingredients

- ½ mango, diced
- ½ cup berries, diced
- 1 peach, diced and skin-removed
- 1 cup plain yogurt or lactose-free yogurt
- ½ cup of ice
- 1 teaspoon stevia (or honey or maple syrup)

<u>Instructions</u>

- Blend all ingredients in a blender and then blend until smooth. Pour into a large glass. Enjoy!

<u>Cooking Tips:</u>

- You can use two tablespoons of agave syrup, honey, or sugar instead of stevia if you can tolerate it.

<u>Diet-related Tips:</u>

- Use honey only if you can tolerate it.
- If you cannot tolerate mango, use papaya instead.

Nutrition Facts

Servings: 1

Amount per serving

Calories	387
	% Daily Value*
Total Fat 4.2g	5%
Saturated Fat 2.7g	13%
Cholesterol 15mg	5%
Sodium 174mg	8%
Total Carbohydrate 69.9g	25%
Dietary Fiber 6.5g	23%
Total Sugars 61.4g	
Protein 17.4g	
Vitamin D 0mcg	0%
Calcium 470mg	36%
Iron 1mg	5%
Potassium 1352mg	29%

PEACH-GINGER SMOOTHIE

A ginger-based smoothie with a fantastic taste!

- Prep Time: 5 minutes
- Serving: 1

Ingredients

- 1 peach, diced and skin-removed
- 1 cup unsweetened almond milk
- 1 tablespoon fresh grated ginger
- 1 teaspoon stevia (or one tablespoon honey or maple syrup)

Instructions

- Blend all ingredients in a blender and then blend until smooth. Pour into a large glass. Enjoy!

Cooking Tips:

- You can use two tablespoons of agave syrup, honey, or sugar instead of stevia if you can tolerate it.

Diet-related Tips:

- Use honey only if you can tolerate it.

Nutrition Facts

Servings: 1

Amount per serving

Calories	208
	% Daily Value*
Total Fat 5.7g	7%
Saturated Fat 3.1g	16%
Cholesterol 20mg	7%
Sodium 127mg	6%
Total Carbohydrate 30.8g	11%
Dietary Fiber 3g	11%
Total Sugars 26.2g	
Protein 9.9g	
Vitamin D 0mcg	0%
Calcium 306mg	24%
Iron 1mg	5%
Potassium 358mg	8%

POMEGRANATE-ANGELICA SMOOTHIE

Enjoy a healthy smoothie with a fantastic sour taste!

- Prep Time: 5 minutes
- Serving: 1-2

Ingredients

- 1 cup pomegranate juice
- ½ cup plain yogurt or lactose-free yogurt
- 1 tablespoon Angelica root powder (optional)

Instructions

- Blend all ingredients in a blender and then blend until smooth. Pour into a large glass. Enjoy!

Cooking Tips:

- You can use one tablespoon of honey or maple syrup for giving sweetness to the smoothie if you can tolerate it.

Diet-related Tips:

- Use honey only if you can tolerate it.
- Make sure you are not eating pomegranate seeds.

Nutrition Facts

Servings: 1

Amount per serving

Calories	**237**
	% Daily Value*
Total Fat 1.5g	2%
Saturated Fat 1.2g	6%
Cholesterol 7mg	2%
Sodium 2421mg	105%
Total Carbohydrate 45.6g	17%
Dietary Fiber 0g	0%
Total Sugars 40.6g	
Protein 7g	
Vitamin D 0mcg	0%
Calcium 246mg	19%
Iron 0mg	1%
Potassium 887mg	19%

APPLE-GINGER SMOOTHIE

A ginger-based smoothie with a fantastic taste!

- Prep Time: 5 minutes
- Serving: 1-2

Ingredients

- 1 apple, diced and skin-removed
- 1 cup unsweetened almond milk
- 3 tablespoons lime juice
- 1 tablespoon fresh grated ginger
- 1 tablespoon honey

Instructions

- Blend all ingredients in a blender and then blend until smooth. Pour into a large glass. Enjoy!

Cooking Tips:

- You can use one tablespoon of maple syrup, or one teaspoon of stevia instead of honey.

Diet-related Tips:

- Use honey only if you can tolerate it.

Bloody Red Drink!

Enjoy a healthy drink with an amazing sour taste!

- Prep Time: 5 minutes
- Serving: 1-2

Ingredients

- 1 cup pomegranate juice
- ½ beet juice
- ½ tablespoon Angelica powder
- 1 tablespoon honey (or maple syrup), to taste

Instructions

- Blend all the ingredients in a blender until smooth. Pour into a large glass. Enjoy!

Cooking Tips:

- You can use one teaspoon of stevia instead of honey or maple syrup.

Diet-related Tips:

- Make sure that you can tolerate beet. Otherwise, remove it from the recipe.
- Use honey only if you can tolerate it.

Nutrition Facts

Servings: 1

Amount per serving

Calories	267

	% Daily Value*
Total Fat 0g	0%
Saturated Fat 0g	0%
Cholesterol 0mg	0%
Sodium 2384mg	104%
Total Carbohydrate 66.3g	24%
Dietary Fiber 0g	0%
Total Sugars 60.3g	
Protein 1.6g	
Vitamin D 0mcg	0%
Calcium 23mg	2%
Iron 0mg	1%
Potassium 611mg	13%

PAPAYA-MANGO-BERRY SMOOTHIE

Enjoy a great combination of papaya and mango in a refreshing smoothie!

- Prep Time: 5-7 minutes
- Serving: 2

Ingredients

- 1 cup mango, diced
- ½ cup mix of berries, diced
- 1 cup papaya chunks
- 1 cup almond milk
- 1 tablespoon honey or maple syrup

Instructions

- Blend all ingredients in a blender and then blend until smooth. Pour into a large glass. Enjoy!

Cooking Tips:

- You can use one teaspoon of stevia instead of honey or maple syrup.

Diet-related Tips:

- Use honey only if you can tolerate it.

Nutrition Facts

Servings: 2

Amount per serving

Calories	398

	% Daily Value*
Total Fat 29g	37%
Saturated Fat 25.5g	127%
Cholesterol 0mg	0%
Sodium 20mg	1%
Total Carbohydrate 38.5g	14%
Dietary Fiber 5.1g	18%
Total Sugars 32g	
Protein 3.9g	
Vitamin D 0mcg	0%
Calcium 39mg	3%
Iron 2mg	13%
Potassium 550mg	12%

Cantaloupe Smoothie

Enjoy a great smoothie with cantaloupe!

- Prep Time: 5 minutes
- Serving: 1-2

Ingredients

- 1 cup cantaloupe, diced
- ½ cup vanilla yogurt or lactose-free yogurt or almond milk
- ½ cup of orange juice
- 1 tablespoon honey (or maple syrup), to taste
- 2 ice cubes

Instructions

- Blend all ingredients in a blender and then blend until smooth. Pour into a large glass. Enjoy!

<u>Cooking Tips:</u>

- You can use 1 teaspoon of stevia instead of honey or maple syrup.

<u>Diet-related Tips:</u>

- Use honey only if you can tolerate it.
- If you cannot tolerate orange juice, simply remove it from the recipe.

Nutrition Facts

Servings: 1

Amount per serving

Calories	260
	% Daily Value*
Total Fat 2.1g	3%
Saturated Fat 1.4g	7%
Cholesterol 7mg	2%
Sodium 113mg	5%
Total Carbohydrate 51.6g	19%
Dietary Fiber 1.7g	6%
Total Sugars 48.5g	
Protein 9.2g	
Vitamin D 0mcg	0%
Calcium 241mg	19%
Iron 2mg	11%
Potassium 962mg	20%

CANTALOUPE-MIX SMOOTHIE

Enjoy a great mix of cantaloupe with mango, lemon, and orange!

- Prep Time: 5-10 minutes
- Serving: 2

<u>Ingredients</u>

- 1 cup cantaloupe, diced
- ½ cup mango, diced

- ½ cup almond milk
- ½ cup of orange juice
- ½ cup mix of berries
- 2 tablespoons lemon
- 1 tablespoon honey (or maple syrup), to taste
- 2 ice cubes

Instructions

- Blend the ingredients in a blender until smooth. Pour into a large glass. Enjoy!

Cooking Tips:

- You can use one teaspoon of stevia instead of honey or maple syrup.

Diet-related Tips:

- Use honey only if you can tolerate it.
- If you cannot tolerate orange juice, remove it from the recipe.
- If you cannot tolerate mango, use papaya instead.

Nutrition Facts

Servings: 2

Amount per serving

Calories	253
	% Daily Value*
Total Fat 14.8g	19%
Saturated Fat 12.8g	64%
Cholesterol 0mg	0%
Sodium 23mg	1%
Total Carbohydrate 32.2g	12%
Dietary Fiber 3.2g	11%
Total Sugars 27.9g	
Protein 3g	
Vitamin D 0mcg	0%
Calcium 26mg	2%
Iron 2mg	12%
Potassium 583mg	12%

APPLESAUCE-AVOCADO SMOOTHIE

Have you tried the taste of applesauce with avocado? Try this smoothie cold!

- Prep Time: 5-7 minutes
- Serving: 1

Ingredients

- 1 cup unsweetened almond
- ½ avocado
- ½ cup applesauce
- ¼ teaspoon ground cinnamon
- ½ cup ice

Instructions

- Blend all ingredients in a blender. Blend the mix until smooth. Pour into a large glass. Enjoy!

Cooking Tips:

- You can use ½ teaspoon of stevia or 1 tablespoon of honey for sweetness.

Nutrition Facts

Servings: 1

Amount per serving

Calories	**299**
	% Daily Value*
Total Fat 23.2g	30%
Saturated Fat 4.4g	22%
Cholesterol 0mg	0%
Sodium 189mg	8%
Total Carbohydrate 24.9g	9%
Dietary Fiber 9.5g	34%
Total Sugars 12.8g	
Protein 3.1g	
Vitamin D 1mcg	7%
Calcium 322mg	25%
Iron 2mg	8%
Potassium 771mg	16%

PINA COLADA SMOOTHIE

A classical gluten-free Mexican smoothie for your parties!

- Prep Time: 5 minutes
- Serving: 1

Ingredients

- 1 cup papaya chunks
- ½ cup unsweetened almond milk
- 1 banana
- ½ teaspoon vanilla extract, to taste
- 1 tablespoon honey, maple syrup or one teaspoon stevia (optional)

Instructions

- Blend all ingredients in a blender and then blend until smooth and creamy. Pour into a large glass. Enjoy!

Cooking Tips:

- For sweetness, you can add stevia, honey, or maple syrup as instructed.

Diet-related Tips:

- Use honey only if you can tolerate it.

Nutrition Facts

Servings: 1

Amount per serving

Calories 348

% Daily Value*

Total Fat 9g	12%
Saturated Fat 6.2g	31%
Cholesterol 0mg	0%
Sodium 98mg	4%
Total Carbohydrate 70.2g	26%
Dietary Fiber 7.7g	28%
Total Sugars 49.4g	
Protein 3.4g	
Vitamin D 1mcg	3%
Calcium 179mg	14%
Iron 4mg	22%
Potassium 783mg	17%

SNACKS

DICED FRUITS

You can dice fresh fruits you can tolerate and use them between your daily main meals. Different types of berries, papaya, honeydew melon, cantaloupe, and banana are some of the best fruits for people with rheumatoid arthritis.

PLAIN YOGURT WITH POACHED FRUITS

Another great snack is mixing plain/vanilla yogurt or lactose-free plain or vanilla yogurt with fruits you can tolerate. As explained, berries, honeydew melon, papaya, cantaloupe, banana, and dark fruits such as red grapes are some of the best fruits for people with rheumatoid arthritis. The following recipe shows how to poach fruits to make a delicious homemade compote.

POACHED FRUIT COMPOTE

It is a great choice that can be consumed by people with rheumatoid arthritis.

- Prep Time: 10 minutes

- Cook Time: 40 Minutes
- Total Time: 50 minutes
- Serving: 6

<u>Ingredients</u>

- 4 peaches, skin removed and thinly sliced
- 1 lb apple, pitted and skin removed
- 1 teaspoon cinnamon powder
- 1 cup honey or maple syrup
- 1 teaspoon vanilla extract

<u>Instructions</u>

1. In a large pot, cook fruits in boiling water over medium heat until softened.
2. In a large bowl, mix well all ingredients (except fruits) together.
3. Pour the syrup over fruits and let the compote be thickened.
4. Pour compote into a jar. Serve hot or cold. Enjoy!

<u>Cooking Tips:</u>

- You can poach fruits with the skin and remove the skin after poaching and before adding syrup to it.
- You can poach other fruits such as pear with the same instructions.
- Make sure you wash fruits thoroughly after peeling them off.

Nutrition Facts

Servings: 6

Amount per serving

Calories | **232**

	% Daily Value*
Total Fat 0.3g	0%
Saturated Fat 0g	0%
Cholesterol 0mg	0%
Sodium 3mg	0%
Total Carbohydrate 61.1g	22%
Dietary Fiber 2.5g	9%
Total Sugars 59.7g	
Protein 1.2g	
Vitamin D 0mcg	0%
Calcium 4mg	0%
Iron 1mg	4%
Potassium 260mg	6%

APPLESAUCE

Applesauce is a fantastic option for people who are following anti-inflammatory diet. You can purchase applesauce from different stores. It is recommended to use organic applesauce, or you can make it at home:

HOMEMADE APPLESAUCE

- Prep Time: 10 minutes
- Cook Time: 30 Minutes
- Total Time: 40 minutes
- Serving: 4

Ingredients

- 6 organic apples, peeled, cored and cubed
- ½ cup boiling water
- ½ teaspoon cinnamon powder
- 4 tablespoons honey
- 2 tablespoons fresh lemon juice

Instructions

1. In a large pot, cook apples with boiling water, lemon juice, cinnamon, and honey over medium-low heat until softened. Remove from heat.
2. You can mash all ingredients by using a fork or blend with a blender or a food processor.
3. Pour applesauce into a suitable container or jar. Serve warm or cold. Enjoy!

<u>Cooking Tips:</u>

- Pink lady apples are preferable for making delicious applesauce.

<u>Diet-related Tips:</u>

- Make sure you wash apples thoroughly after peeling them off.
- If you cannot tolerate honey well, you may add one tablespoon of Stevia instead.

Nutrition Facts

Servings: 4

Amount per serving

Calories	**223**
	% Daily Value*
Total Fat 0.7g	1%
Saturated Fat 0.1g	0%
Cholesterol 0mg	0%
Sodium 5mg	0%
Total Carbohydrate 58.9g	21%
Dietary Fiber 8.1g	29%
Total Sugars 47.5g	
Protein 1g	
Vitamin D 0mcg	0%
Calcium 3mg	0%
Iron 2mg	8%
Potassium 368mg	8%

AVOCADO DIP

A modified avocado dip recipe is a great snack candidate for people with rheumatoid arthritis.

- Prep Time: 5 minutes
- Cook Time: 0 minutes
- Total Time: 5 minutes
- Serving: 4-6

Ingredients

- 6 avocados, peeled
- ½ tablespoon extra virgin olive oil
- ¼ cup chopped fresh cilantro
- 2 tablespoons fresh lime juice
- 1 teaspoon fresh lemon juice

Instructions

1. In a large bowl, mash avocados with a fork.
2. Add extra virgin olive oil and other ingredients into it.
3. Enjoy!

Cooking Tips:

- If you can tolerate a few tomatoes and onions, cube them and then add them into your guacamole.

Nutrition Facts

Servings: 6

Amount per serving

Calories	422
	% Daily Value*
Total Fat 40.4g	52%
Saturated Fat 8.4g	42%
Cholesterol 0mg	0%
Sodium 207mg	9%
Total Carbohydrate 18g	7%
Dietary Fiber 13.5g	48%
Total Sugars 1.2g	
Protein 3.9g	
Vitamin D 0mcg	0%
Calcium 26mg	2%
Iron 1mg	7%
Potassium 988mg	21%

HOMEMADE HUMMUS

A healthy and tasty middle-eastern snack. An excellent option for vegetarians and for people with rheumatoid arthritis during the remission period.

- Prep Time: 5 minutes
- Cook Time: 60 minutes
- Total Time: 65 minutes
- Serving: 4

<u>Ingredients</u>

- ¼ lb dried chickpeas (soaked in water for one night)
- 1½ tablespoon tahini
- 1 tablespoon lemon juice
- 2 tablespoons extra virgin olive oil, divided
- ¼ teaspoon cumin
- 1 tablespoon water
- 1 teaspoon baking soda (optional)
- 1 teaspoon paprika powder (optional)

<u>Instructions</u>

1. First, people with rheumatoid arthritis need to soak the chickpeas overnight in water and optionally add baking soda to the water.
2. Cook your chickpeas in a large pot with water, over medium heat for about one hour. Check if chickpeas cooked well by crushing one of them with a fork in your hand.
3. When chickpeas cooked, drain them and put them in a blender.

4. Add 1 tablespoon of extra virgin olive oil, lemon juice, tahini, and cumin powder to the blender. Blend until your hummus gets a soft, creamy texture equally.
5. Sprinkle with one tablespoon extra virgin olive oil or paprika powder (optional).
6. Serve immediately or fridge it.

Cooking Tips:

- You can serve hummus, hot or cold.

Diet-related Tips:

- Eat hummus in moderation when you are in remission.

Nutrition Facts

Servings: 4

Amount per serving

Calories	198
	% Daily Value*
Total Fat 11.8g	15%
Saturated Fat 1.6g	8%
Cholesterol 0mg	0%
Sodium 305mg	13%
Total Carbohydrate 18.5g	7%
Dietary Fiber 5.5g	20%
Total Sugars 3.1g	
Protein 6.5g	
Vitamin D 0mcg	0%
Calcium 56mg	4%
Iron 2mg	13%
Potassium 279mg	6%

TOFU

Tofu is a fantastic snack option for people with rheumatoid arthritis in general. It is based on soy milk and is rich in calcium and Iron, needed for most patients. Here is a sample recipe of a snack with Tofu:

AVOCADO TOFU TOAST

Enjoy a healthy and rich daily snack!

- Prep Time: 10 minutes
- Cook Time: 35 minutes
- Total Time: 45 minutes
- Serving: 4

Ingredients

- 1½ cup firm tofu, pressed and drained
- 1 avocado, cubed
- 1 tablespoon extra virgin olive oil
- Pepper, to taste

Instructions

1. Preheat your oven to 400 °F.
2. Choose a baking sheet, cover it with parchment paper or spray extra virgin olive oil. Cut tofu-like cubes of 1.5 inches and spray extra virgin olive oil on it.
3. Let it bake for 15 minutes until golden brown and crispy. Flip tofu and cook for another 10 minutes. Remove from the oven. Let it rest for 10 minutes.
4. Cube avocado on a plate and add Pepper.
5. Mix the tofu with avocado in a bowl. Enjoy!

Cooking Tips:

- You may want to add one tablespoon of lemon juice to create another great taste.

ALMOND BUTTER SANDWICH

Almond butter is a fantastic source of fiber and magnesium for people with rheumatoid arthritis. It is recommended to use smooth almond butter.

- Prep Time: 5 minutes
- Total Time: 5 minutes
- Serving: 1

Ingredients

- 2 slices of gluten-free bread
- 1 tablespoon organic smooth almond butter

Instructions

1. Spread one piece of bread with almond butter.
2. Toast and enjoy!

Cooking Tips:

- Remember to use smooth almond butter.

Nutrition Facts

Servings: 1

Amount per serving

Calories 313

% Daily Value*

Total Fat 17.7g 23%

Saturated Fat 1.9g 9%

Cholesterol 0mg 0%

Sodium 341mg 15%

Total Carbohydrate 32.3g 12%

Dietary Fiber 5.2g 19%

Total Sugars 4.2g

Protein 8.8g

Vitamin D 0mcg 0%

Calcium 156mg 12%

Iron 3mg 16%

Potassium 280mg 6%

GLUTEN-FREE MUFFINS

You may eat different types of muffins, but you have to make sure about the ingredients. The muffin should not be made with fruits you cannot tolerate. Moreover, try not to eat muffins that are made with whole-wheat flour. If you are gluten-intolerant or suffering from RA, you can make your muffins at home:

- Prep Time: 15 minutes
- Cook Time: 45 minutes
- Total Time: 60 minutes
- Serving: 5-10 (10 Muffins)

<u>Ingredients</u>

- 2 tablespoons extra virgin olive oil or avocado oil
- 2½ cups almond flour, blanched
- 3 large organic free-range eggs
- ¼ cup organic maple syrup
- 2 teaspoons vanilla extract
- ¼ cup banana, mashed
- 1 teaspoon lemon juice
- ¾ teaspoon baking soda

- ¼ teaspoon cinnamon powder

Instructions

1. Preheat your oven to 375 °F.
2. In a large bowl, mix almond flour, cinnamon, and baking soda. Whisk well.
3. In another bowl, add extra virgin olive oil, vanilla extract, eggs, ripe banana, maple syrup, and lemon juice. Whisk well.
4. Mix the two bowls and stir well with a wooden spoon until flour mixed well with other ingredients.
5. Prepare ten muffin cups. Pour them to the top and then bake for 15 minutes.
6. To avoid browning quickly, loosely cover muffins with an aluminum foil. Cook for another 15 minutes.
7. Put a toothpick in a muffin to check if it cooks well or not. If cooked well, the toothpick should not stick to the muffin.
8. Remove from the oven. Let the muffins cool for 15 more minutes. Enjoy!

Cooking Tips:

- You need to use finely grounded skin-removed flour.

Nutrition Facts

Servings: 10

Amount per serving

Calories	366
	% Daily Value*
Total Fat 30.7g	39%
Saturated Fat 2.9g	14%
Cholesterol 65mg	22%
Sodium 242mg	11%
Total Carbohydrate 16.1g	6%
Dietary Fiber 5.1g	18%
Total Sugars 7.8g	
Protein 12.8g	
Vitamin D 0mcg	0%
Calcium 132mg	10%
Iron 2mg	11%
Potassium 31mg	1%

AVOCADO TUNA TOAST

A very fast sandwich you can prepare at home.

- Prep Time: 10 minutes
- Cook Time: 0 minutes
- Total Time: 10 minutes
- Serving: 4

Ingredients

- 2 avocados
- 2 tablespoons organic low-sodium mayonnaise
- 1 teaspoon cumin powder
- 1 can of tuna in olive oil or water
- ¼ cup apple, chopped and peeled off
- 4 whole grain toasts or any gluten-free bread
- Pepper to taste (optional)

Instructions

1. Choose a small bowl. Mix tuna with smashed avocado with mayo, cumin powder, peeled off apple (cut into small pieces), and pepper (optional).
2. Place tuna mix on two toast slices. Cover with other slices.
3. Toast and enjoy!

Cooking Tips:

- You can make this sandwich without mayonnaise sauce, as well.

Nutrition Facts

Servings: 4

Amount per serving

Calories 386

% Daily Value*

Total Fat 26.7g	34%
Saturated Fat 5.2g	26%
Cholesterol 17mg	6%
Sodium 268mg	12%
Total Carbohydrate 23.3g	8%
Dietary Fiber 7.7g	27%
Total Sugars 3g	
Protein 15.8g	
Vitamin D 0mcg	0%
Calcium 45mg	3%
Iron 2mg	11%
Potassium 689mg	15%

GINGER BISCUITS

Ginger is rich in potassium and vitamin B6 with excellent anti-inflammatory properties. Hence, ginger-based snacks are great snack options for people with rheumatoid arthritis.

GLUTEN-FREE GINGER BISCUITS

Enjoy making a gluten-free, dairy-free ginger biscuit in your home.

- Prep Time: 15 minutes
- Cook Time: 20 minutes
- Total Time: 35 minutes
- Serving: 4-6

<u>Ingredients</u>

- ¾ cup shortening or half a cup + 1 tablespoon extra virgin olive oil
- 2 cups gluten-free flour or grated almond flour
- 2 tablespoons honey
- 1 organic, free-range egg
- 2 teaspoons baking soda
- ¼ cup molasses

- 1½ teaspoons freshly grated ginger
- 1 teaspoon cinnamon powder

<u>Instructions</u>

1. In a large bowl, mix oil (or shortening), sugar, molasses, and egg.
2. In another large bowl, mix flour, ginger, baking soda, and cinnamon.
3. Slowly combine ingredients of both bowls until making a soft dough.
4. Let the dough rest for 45 minutes.
5. Preheat oven to 375°F.
6. Roll the dough and make 2-inch (5cm) balls. Pour honey on dough balls.
7. Use cookie sheets with parchment paper. Put balls on cooking sheets and bake for 12-15 minutes until seeing cracks and until having a light brown color.
8. Remove from the oven and cool biscuits for five minutes. Enjoy!

<u>Cooking Tips:</u>

- Shortening gives you a better ginger biscuit texture. However, some patients may not tolerate it well. Alternatively, use olive oil.
- If you cannot tolerate honey, you can use a little bit of sugar or maple syrup.
- You can substitute ¼ cup of molasses with ¼ cup maple syrup.

<u>Diet-related Tips:</u>

- Do not use molasses if you cannot tolerate it. Instead, use maple syrup.

ZUCCHINI CHIPS

Zucchini chips are a healthy, low-calorie snack for people with rheumatoid arthritis with lots of crunchiness as well as vitamin C and B6!

- Prep Time: 20 minutes
- Cook Time: 90 minutes
- Total Time: 110 minutes
- Serving: 2-4

Ingredients

- 2 zucchinis, sliced thin
- 1 tablespoon extra virgin olive oil
- ¼ teaspoon cumin powder (optional)
- Pepper, to taste

Instructions

1- Slice zucchinis lengthwise and thin by a slicer.
2- Take out the moisture from zucchinis using clean paper towels. Hold and press down paper towels on zucchinis.
3- Preheat the over to 250 °F.

4- Spray olive oil on parchment papers and then, place zucchinis on them.

5- Spray or pour olive oil on top of zucchinis as well. Sprinkle pepper and cumin powder (optional).

6- Bake zucchinis for about 80-90 minutes until golden.

7- Remove from the oven. Dry zucchinis with a paper towel. Enjoy!

<u>Cooking Tips:</u>

- You can also fry zucchinis in a large pan by extra virgin olive oil over low heat or microwave it. For more crispiness, you may need to broil fried zucchinis.

<u>Diet-related Tips:</u>

- Use this recipe only if you can tolerate zucchini as a nightshade.

Nutrition Facts
Servings: 2

Amount per serving
Calories   **95**

	% Daily Value*
Total Fat 7.4g	10%
Saturated Fat 1.1g	5%
Cholesterol 0mg	0%
Sodium 20mg	1%
Total Carbohydrate 7.2g	3%
Dietary Fiber 2.3g	8%
Total Sugars 3.6g	
Protein 2.5g	
Vitamin D 0mcg	0%
Calcium 32mg	2%
Iron 1mg	5%
Potassium 526mg	11%

DRINKS

RECOMMENDED HOT BEVERAGES

Some hot beverages recommended for people with rheumatoid arthritis are:

- <u>Green Tea:</u> is another excellent choice for people with rheumatoid arthritis. It includes polyphenol antioxidants such as epigallocatechin gallate (EGCG), a type of catechin that protects cells from damages and can reduce inflammation that can help soothe RA symptoms. It can also help inhibit bacterial growth, which lowers the risks of getting infections. Moreover, green tea contains less caffeine than regular coffee. However, it could give you a similar mood.

- <u>Decaffeinated black tea:</u> if you would like to have earl gray, English breakfast, or any types of black tea, it is better to drink decaffeinated kinds, especially if you are experiencing a flare-up. If you are in remission, take caffeinated black tea in moderation. As cinnamon has anti-inflammatory properties, it is a great idea to pour a little bit of cinnamon powder in your black tea.

- <u>Peppermint Tea:</u> this herbal tea is an excellent choice for people with rheumatoid arthritis as it has properties that can soothe your inflammation.

- <u>Ziziphora/Oregano/Thyme Tea:</u> This herbal tea is recommended for people with rheumatoid arthritis. Ziziphora is the name of a mountain plant from the Lamiaceae group, similar to Thyme. It has flavonoids with anti-inflammatory properties. Oregano contains great antioxidants such as Carvacrol and Thymol that can reduce the risk of virus activities. Studies have shown excellent anti-inflammatory properties of oregano. Thyme tea is also great for people with rheumatoid arthritis. It has antioxidants and antimicrobial properties with valuable sources of Iron. Thyme can also be used in foods as a great seasoning. You can pour one tablespoon of Ziziphora or Oregano or Thyme in a cup of boiling water and enjoy drinking this fantastic tea after 8-10 minutes.

- <u>Turmeric and Ginger Tea:</u> both turmeric and ginger are fantastic for people with rheumatoid arthritis. Turmeric and Ginger have been used widely in ancient medicine. They use turmeric and ginger as medicines and for better digestion. Turmeric is high in antioxidants that can protect your cells from damaging and reduces the risks of getting infections. Curcumin in turmeric is a great anti-inflammatory ingredient. Ginger also has strong anti-inflammatory properties that can help reduce inflammation in the GI tract.
    - For making a great tea, add ½ teaspoon of ground turmeric and ½ teaspoon of freshly grated ginger in 2 cups of boiling water and enjoy your drink after 12-15 minutes. You can add 1-teaspoon honey or maple syrup to your tea if you can tolerate it. One of the delicious hot beverages you can make with Turmeric and Ginger is called Golden Milk.
    - Golden Milk: mix ½ cup of unsweetened almond milk, one teaspoon turmeric, ½ teaspoon of freshly grated ginger, ½ teaspoon of cinnamon powder, and one teaspoon of honey or maple syrup (optional: if you can tolerate) in a small pot and boil. After boiling, simmer for 5 minutes until flavors over low heat.
- <u>Ginger-Mint Tea:</u> you can benefit from both ginger and mint properties by making this great tea. Mint

has menthol, which helps reduce inflammation in the gut.

Boil 10-15 mint leaves with one tablespoon of lemon juice and ½ teaspoon of freshly grated ginger and 2 cups of water in a small pot. Remove from heat, wait for three more minutes and add one tablespoon honey or maple syrup (optional: if you can tolerate) for sweetness if you want.

- <u>Slippery Elm Tea:</u> recent studies showed that slippery elm bark could soothe inflammation and might be an excellent drink for patients with autoimmune diseases. Pour one tablespoon of slippery elm in a cup of boiling water and enjoy drinking after 10 minutes.
- <u>Calendula Tea:</u> this tea is known for helping people with peptic ulcers, reflux, and inflammation. It may soothe inflammation and irritation as it has anti-inflammatory and wound-healing properties. Pour 1 tablespoon of dried calendula in a cup of boiling water and enjoy drinking after 10-12 minutes.
- <u>Milk?:</u> Generally speaking, people with rheumatoid arthritis cannot use milk. However, some researches show anti-inflammatory properties of milk. Hence, always consult with your doctor if you want to drink milk. If you are in remission, it is recommended to consume unsweetened almond milk. You can also use soy milk during remissions, but make sure you are using a Non-GMO type. Always check your intolerance level first.
- <u>Coffee:</u> in general, coffee might be fine for people with RA. However, some studies say coffee can increase the risk of RA and some studies explain only decaffeinated coffee is troublesome. In general, it is

recommended to avoid decaffeinated coffee and reduce your regular coffee intake during remissions. During flares, avoid drinking coffee. Remember to consult with your doctor or nutritionist about drinking coffee.

- Hot chocolate (especially hot dark chocolate) is another drink that has anti-inflammatory properties and might be consumed only if you can tolerate it.

RECOMMENDED COLD BEVERAGES

Some recommended cold beverages for people with rheumatoid arthritis are as below:

- <u>Water:</u> The best drink for people with rheumatoid arthritis is water. Try drinking at least 8-10 glasses of water each day, especially if you are experiencing a flare-up, which helps reduce your inflammation.
  - o Some patients experienced better feelings of consuming alkaline water with 9.5 pH. Alkaline water is water with a pH of more than 7 (normal). As it has a higher pH than regular water, some claim that it can balance body pH level. Most soda drinks in the market have acidic properties (pH smaller than 7). Ionized alkaline water can increase hydration as ionization may reduce the size of molecular clusters of water. Some experts also claimed that as active oxygen in water is a free radical, it might damage healthy tissues. Alkaline water may neutralize active oxygen and avoid those damaging healthy tissues.

- <u>Do not drink</u> soda, carbonated beverages, and diet beverages. These drinks may activate your symptoms.
- <u>Fruit Juices:</u> Fruit juices are excellent sources of vitamins for people with rheumatoid arthritis. Juicing is essential for people with rheumatoid arthritis, as many of them cannot digest fibers in foods and fruits easily. Hence, they can boost their nutrient intake by juicing. However, people with rheumatoid arthritis need to consume fruits with no added sugars or any types of artificial sweeteners:
  - It is recommended to avoid add sugar or any artificial sweeteners to juices. If you can tolerate honey, maple syrup, or stevia, you can add them to your juice.
  - The best fruit juice that can be consumed in moderation are:

    Aloe Vera, Papaya, Berries, Honeydew Melon, Banana, Carrot, Cantaloupe, Squash, Pumpkin, Cucumber (peeled), and dark fruits such as dark grapes.
  - You may want to try other fruit juices such as apple, peach, mango or pear. You may also juice vegetables such as celery, broccoli and spinach. Always start consuming less and check your tolerance level.
  - Many people with rheumatoid arthritis can't tolerate tomato juice and other nightshade's juice. Ask your doctor and check your tolerance before consumption.

  It is better to purchase organic fruits and always correctly wash fruits first, even if you know that you want to remove their skin.

- <u>Alcohol:</u> alcohol needs to be avoided as much as possible by rheumatoid arthritis patients.

- <u>Alcohol:</u> alcohol needs to be avoided as much as

CHAPTER 6. MEAL PLANNING

This chapter provides you with an example of a biweekly meal plans. It can give you an idea of how to create your biweekly plans for remission and flare-up periods.

Here are some of the essential tips you need to remember when you want to make your meal plan for remission periods:

COOKING PLAN FOR REMISSION PERIODS:

- Try varieties of foods, but always eat and drink healthy foods.
- If you are lactose-intolerant, try alternative products explained in this book.
- If you are gluten-intolerant, try alternative products explained in this book.
- When you are in remission, it does not mean that you can eat everything. There are still some triggering foods to avoid as they can wake up flares. Always make your meal plan based on your health conditions and non-triggering foods that can be well-tolerated by you.
- If you are sensitive to seafood, you can substitute seafood with other foods with healthy fat and protein sources. Many non-seafood cooking recipes are available in this book.
- Remember that it is recommended to eat six portions a day. Hence, you can have breakfast, snack (between breakfast and lunch), lunch, snack (between lunch and dinner), dinner, and snack (between dinner and your sleep time). You can use appetizers, snacks,

desserts, and snack recipes in this book for snack portions. Alternatively, you can have soups or salads as before-lunch or before-dinner snacks.

Here is an example of a biweekly meal plan for remission Periods:

Week-1:	Week-2:
Monday	Monday
Breakfast: Avocado Egg Breakfast Toast **Snack-1:** Zucchini Chips **Lunch:** Chicken Kebab (From Last Night) **Snack-2:** Banana Milkshake **Dinner:** Grilled Honey Salmon **Snack-3:** Diced Fruits **Drinks:** Peppermint Tea	**Breakfast:** Egg Tacos with Avocado **Snack-1:** Gluten-Free Crackers **Lunch:** Chicken Stroganoff (From Last Night) **Snack-2:** Cooler Drink or Almond Butter Toast **Dinner:** Lemon Steamed Halibut with Brown Rice **Snack-3:** Apple Ginger Sundae **Drinks:** Earl Gray Tea, Green Tea
Tuesday	Tuesday
Breakfast: Almond Butter Banana Sandwich **Snack-1:** Gluten-Free Ginger Biscuit **Lunch:** Grilled Honey Salmon and **Snack-2:** Avocado Smoothie **Dinner:** Stracciatella Soup **Snack-3:** Applesauce **Drinks:** Black Tea, Green Tea	**Breakfast:** Fruit Salad with Almond Milk **Snack-1:** Avocado Dip **Lunch:** Lemon Steamed Halibut with Brown Rice **Snack-2:** Banana Cinnamon Smoothie **Dinner:** Classic Tuna Pasta Salad or Butternut Squash Soup **Snack-3:** Pomegranate Angelica Drink **Drinks:** Decaffeinated Coffee, Peppermint Tea
Wednesday	Wednesday
Breakfast: Apple Cinnamon Oatmeal **Snack-1:** Tofu Toast **Lunch:** Stracciatella Soup **Snack-2:** Cantaloupe Smoothie **Dinner:** Balsamic Peach Pork **Snack-3:** Poached Fruit Compote **Drinks:** Coffee, Peppermint Tea	**Breakfast:** Oatmeal **Snack-1:** Guacamole-Like Snack **Lunch:** Classic Tuna Pasta Salad or Butternut Squash Soup **Snack-2:** Banana Milkshake **Dinner:** Pumpkin Soup **Snack-3:** Cantaloupe Mix Smoothie **Drinks:** Coffee, Oregano Tea
Thursday	Thursday
Breakfast: Gluten-Free Fluffy Pancakes **Snack-1:** Fruit Bowl from berries **Lunch:** Balsamic Peach Pork **Snack-2:** Peach Mango Banana Smoothie **Dinner:** Thunfisch Pizza and/or Butternut Squash Soup **Snack-3:** Gluten-Free Apple Pie **Drinks:** Black Tea with Cinnamon, Ginger Mint Tea	**Breakfast:** Baked Apple **Snack-1:** Avocado Bagel **Lunch:** Pumpkin Soup **Snack-2:** Baba Ghanoush **Dinner:** Grilled Ostrich Meat Kebab with Brown Rice **Snack-3:** Carrot Juice with Mango Ice Cream **Drinks:** Earl Grey Tea, Ginger Mint Tea
Friday	Friday
Breakfast: Two Poached Eggs with Toasts **Snack-1:** Almond Butter Sandwich **Lunch:** Thunfisch Pizza and/or Butternut Squash Soup **Snack-2:** Banana Cinnamon Smoothie	**Breakfast:** Almond Butter Honey Banana Toast **Snack-1:** Applesauce **Lunch:** Grilled Ostrich Meat Kebab with Brown Rice **Snack-2:** Carrot Avocado Salad **Dinner:** Chicken Pizza

Dinner: Chicken Zucchini Stew with Chicken Broth **Snack-3:** Diced Fruits such as Papaya **Drinks:** Coffee, Ziziphora Tea	**Snack-3:** Warm Apple Crumble **Drinks:** Green Tea
Saturday	Saturday
Breakfast: Avocado Bagel **Snack-1:** Poached Fruits with Plain Yogurt **Lunch:** Chicken Zucchini Stew with Chicken Broth **Snack-2:** Butter Lettuce Salad **Dinner:** Hungarian Goulash **Snack-3:** Lemon Sorbet or a Fruit Juice **Drinks:** Turmeric Ginger Tea	**Breakfast:** Egg Salmon Avocado **Snack-1:** Tofu Toast **Lunch:** Chicken Pizza **Snack-2:** Applesauce Avocado Smoothie **Dinner:** Chicken & Shrimp Teriyaki **Snack-3:** Gluten-free Crackers **Drinks:** Turmeric Ginger Tea
Sunday	Sunday
Breakfast: Smoothie Bowl with Almond Milk **Snack-1:** Gluten-Free Crackers **Lunch:** Hungarian Goulash with Bone Broth **Snack-2:** Hummus **Dinner:** Chicken Stroganoff **Snack-3:** Avocado Peach Popsicle **Drinks:** Slippery Elm Tea	**Breakfast:** Zucchini Bread Oatmeal **Snack-1:** Gluten-Free Ginger Biscuit **Lunch:** Chicken & Shrimp Teriyaki **Snack-2:** Apple Pear Salad **Dinner:** Ginger Sticky Pork **Snack-3:** Pear Cake Sundae **Drinks:** Black Tea, Calendula Tea

Here are some of the critical points you need to remember when you want to make your meal plan for flare-up periods:

COOKING PLAN FOR FLARE-UP PERIODS

- You have to limit yourself to non-triggering healthy food recipes.
- It is recommended to avoid consuming lactose and gluten during flares.
- Remember: when you are in a flare, you have to put more non-triggering soups, juices, and broth in your meal plan.
- Always make your meal plan based on your health conditions and non-triggering foods that can be well-tolerated by you.
- During flares, stick to your meal plan and modify it only if you found any intolerable foods/ingredients.

- Put more foods with anti-inflammatory herbs and spices such as turmeric and ginger in your flare-up meal plan.
- Drink safe anti-inflammatory herbal teas such as peppermint and green tea during flare-up periods.
- If you are sensitive to seafood, you can substitute seafood with other foods with healthy fat and protein sources. Many non-seafood cooking recipes provided for you in this book.
- Remember that it is recommended to eat six portions a day instead of three portions. Hence, you can have breakfast, snack (between breakfast and lunch), lunch, snack (between lunch and dinner), dinner, and snack (between dinner and your sleep time). You can use appetizers, snacks, desserts, and snack recipes in this book for snack portions. Alternatively, you can have soups or salads as before-lunch or before-dinner snacks.
- If you have issues in making an effective meal plan for your flare-up periods, ask support from a nutritionist or a dietitian. Here is an example of a biweekly flare-up meal plan:

Week-1:	Week-2:
Monday	Monday
Breakfast: Avocado + 2 Poached Eggs **Snack-1:** Zucchini Salad **Lunch:** Chicken Kebab with Brown Rice (From Last Night) **Snack-2:** Carrot Juice **Dinner:** Boiled Salmon / Carrot Potato Soup **Snack-3:** Diced Non-Triggering Fruits **Drinks:** Peppermint Tea	**Breakfast:** Two Poached Eggs with Avocado **Snack-1:** Avocado Dip **Lunch:** Chicken Noodle Soup (From Last Night) **Snack-2:** Cooler Drink **Dinner:** Lemon Steamed Halibut with Brown Rice **Snack-3:** Ginger Fruit Sherbet (Sweetened by Stevia) **Drinks:** Black Tea, Green Tea
Tuesday	Tuesday
Breakfast: Smooth Almond Butter Banana Sandwich **Snack-1:** Gluten-Free Ginger Biscuit **Lunch:** Boiled Salmon / Carrot Potato Soup **Snack-2:** Cantaloupe or Berry Juice **Dinner:** Turkey Pot Pie Soup **Snack-3:** Applesauce **Drinks:** Black Tea, Green Tea	**Breakfast:** Fruit Salad **Snack-1:** Oatmeal or Firm Tofu **Lunch:** Lemon Steamed Halibut with Brown Rice **Snack-2:** Carrot Juice **Dinner:** Classic Tuna Pasta Salad **Snack-3:** Pomegranate Angelica Drink **Drinks:** Peppermint Tea
Wednesday	Wednesday
Breakfast: Oatmeal or Fruit Bowl with Berries **Snack-1:** Firm Tofu Toast **Lunch:** Turkey Pot Pie Soup **Snack-2:** Honeydew Melon Juice **Dinner:** Carrot Avocado Salad **Snack-3:** Poached Fruit Compote (e.g., Peeled Apple) **Drinks:** Green Tea, Peppermint Tea	**Breakfast:** Oatmeal or Fruit Bowl with Berries **Snack-1:** Guacamole-Like Snack **Lunch:** Classic Tuna Pasta Salad **Snack-2:** Diced Banana **Dinner:** Pumpkin Soup **Snack-3:** Cantaloupe Juice **Drinks:** Green Tea, Peppermint Tea
Thursday	Thursday
Breakfast: Two Poached Eggs with Toasts **Snack-1:** Diced Fruits **Lunch:** Carrot Avocado Salad **Snack-2:** Applesauce Avocado Smoothie (Dairy-Free) **Dinner:** Butternut Squash Soup **Snack-3:** Cantaloupe or Watermelon Juice **Drinks:** Black Tea, Ginger Mint Tea	**Breakfast:** Baked Apple **Snack-1:** Smooth Almond Butter Sandwich **Lunch:** Pumpkin Soup **Snack-2:** Poached Egg Avocado White Pita **Dinner:** Turkey Zucchini Noodles **Snack-3:** Carrot Juice **Drinks:** Earl Grey Tea, Ginger Mint Tea
Friday	Friday
Breakfast: Avocado + Gluten-Free Bagel **Snack-1:** Almond Butter Sandwich **Lunch:** Butternut Squash Soup **Snack-2:** Applesauce **Dinner:** Chicken Zucchini Stew with Chicken Broth **Snack-3:** Diced Fruits such as Papaya	**Breakfast:** Almond Butter Honey Banana Toast **Snack-1:** Applesauce **Lunch:** Turkey Zucchini Noodles **Snack-2:** Carrot Avocado Salad **Dinner:** Butternut Squash Soup **Snack-3:** Lemon Sorbet **Drinks:** Peppermint Tea, Green Tea

Drinks: Peppermint Tea	
Saturday	Saturday
Breakfast: Smooth Almond Butter Banana Sandwich **Snack-1:** Poached Fruits (Unsweetened or with Stevia) **Lunch:** Chicken Zucchini Stew with Chicken Broth **Snack-2:** Ginger Cool Drink **Dinner:** Boiled Salmon or Trout **Snack-3:** Lemon Sorbet **Drinks:** Turmeric Ginger Tea	**Breakfast:** 2 Poached Eggs with Avocado **Snack-1:** Firm Tofu Toast **Lunch:** Butternut Squash Soup **Snack-2:** Papaya Dices **Dinner:** Lemon Shrimp with Brown Rice **Snack-3:** Gluten-free crackers **Drinks:** Turmeric Ginger Tea
Sunday	Sunday
Breakfast: Smoothie Bowl with Almond Milk **Snack-1:** Gluten-Free Rice Crackers or Applesauce **Lunch:** Boiled Salmon or Trout **Snack-2:** Guacamole Like Snack **Dinner:** Chicken Noodle Soup **Snack-3:** Popsicle from a Non-triggering Fruit **Drinks:** Green Tea	**Breakfast:** Zucchini Bread Oatmeal **Snack-1:** Gluten-Free Ginger Biscuit **Lunch:** Lemon Shrimp with Brown Rice **Snack-2:** Apple Pear Salad **Dinner:** Stracciatella Soup + Zucchini Salad **Snack-3:** Popsicle from Berries **Drinks:** Black Tea, Peppermint Tea

BIWEEKLY COOKING PLAN – BLANK

This section gives you two free blank meal plan tables that can be filled by you if you want to create your biweekly meal plans.

Biweekly Meal Plan	
Week-1:	**Week-2:**
Monday	Monday
Breakfast: **Snack-1:** **Lunch:** **Snack-2:** **Dinner:** **Snack-3:** **Drinks:**	**Breakfast:** **Snack-1:** **Lunch:** **Snack-2:** **Dinner:** **Snack-3:** **Drinks:**
Tuesday	Tuesday
Breakfast: **Snack-1:** **Lunch:** **Snack-2:** **Dinner:** **Snack-3:** **Drinks:**	**Breakfast:** **Snack-1:** **Lunch:** **Snack-2:** **Dinner:** **Snack-3:** **Drinks:**
Wednesday	Wednesday
Breakfast: **Snack-1:** **Lunch:** **Snack-2:** **Dinner:** **Snack-3:** **Drinks:**	**Breakfast:** **Snack-1:** **Lunch:** **Snack-2:** **Dinner:** **Snack-3:** **Drinks:**
Thursday	Thursday
Breakfast: **Snack-1:** **Lunch:** **Snack-2:** **Dinner:** **Snack-3:** **Drinks:**	**Breakfast:** **Snack-1:** **Lunch:** **Snack-2:** **Dinner:** **Snack-3:** **Drinks:**
Friday	Friday
Breakfast: **Snack-1:** **Lunch:** **Snack-2:** **Dinner:** **Snack-3:** **Drinks:**	**Breakfast:** **Snack-1:** **Lunch:** **Snack-2:** **Dinner:** **Snack-3:** **Drinks:**
Saturday	Saturday
Breakfast: **Snack-1:** **Lunch:** **Snack-2:** **Dinner:** **Snack-3:** **Drinks:**	**Breakfast:** **Snack-1:** **Lunch:** **Snack-2:** **Dinner:** **Snack-3:** **Drinks:**
Sunday	Sunday
Breakfast: **Snack-1:** **Lunch:** **Snack-2:** **Dinner:** **Snack-3:** **Drinks:**	**Breakfast:** **Snack-1:** **Lunch:** **Snack-2:** **Dinner:** **Snack-3:** **Drinks:**

Biweekly Meal Plan	
Week-1:	**Week-2:**
Monday	Monday
Breakfast: **Snack-1:** **Lunch:** **Snack-2:** **Dinner:** **Snack-3:** **Drinks:**	**Breakfast:** **Snack-1:** **Lunch:** **Snack-2:** **Dinner:** **Snack-3:** **Drinks:**
Tuesday	Tuesday
Breakfast: **Snack-1:** **Lunch:** **Snack-2:** **Dinner:** **Snack-3:** **Drinks:**	**Breakfast:** **Snack-1:** **Lunch:** **Snack-2:** **Dinner:** **Snack-3:** **Drinks:**
Wednesday	Wednesday
Breakfast: **Snack-1:** **Lunch:** **Snack-2:** **Dinner:** **Snack-3:** **Drinks:**	**Breakfast:** **Snack-1:** **Lunch:** **Snack-2:** **Dinner:** **Snack-3:** **Drinks:**
Thursday	Thursday
Breakfast: **Snack-1:** **Lunch:** **Snack-2:** **Dinner:** **Snack-3:** **Drinks:**	**Breakfast:** **Snack-1:** **Lunch:** **Snack-2:** **Dinner:** **Snack-3:** **Drinks:**
Friday	Friday
Breakfast: **Snack-1:** **Lunch:** **Snack-2:** **Dinner:** **Snack-3:** **Drinks:**	**Breakfast:** **Snack-1:** **Lunch:** **Snack-2:** **Dinner:** **Snack-3:** **Drinks:**
Saturday	Saturday
Breakfast: **Snack-1:** **Lunch:** **Snack-2:** **Dinner:** **Snack-3:** **Drinks:**	**Breakfast:** **Snack-1:** **Lunch:** **Snack-2:** **Dinner:** **Snack-3:** **Drinks:**
Sunday	Sunday
Breakfast: **Snack-1:** **Lunch:** **Snack-2:** **Dinner:** **Snack-3:** **Drinks:**	**Breakfast:** **Snack-1:** **Lunch:** **Snack-2:** **Dinner:** **Snack-3:** **Drinks:**

This book aimed to provide you with useful information about rheumatoid arthritis diet healthy nutritional choices, food preparation, how to cook for rheumatoid arthritis patients who needs to follow anti-inflammatory diet and essential dietary tips you need to know to effectively manage rheumatoid arthritis. It also guided you through meal planning and how to create biweekly meal plans.

Comprehensive lists of foods to avoid and foods to each for people who want to follow the anti-inflammatory RA diet presented in Chapter 2, and Chapter 3 and 4 suggested essential tips for food preparation and meal planning. You learned more than 120 different cooking recipes presented in Chapter 5 of this book, including cooking tips and diet-related tips.

Chapter 6 presented biweekly meal plan samples. The blanked biweekly cooking plan tables in this chapter can be used by you to write your own meal plans. Remember that it is always essential to talk to your doctor or nutritionist about suggested foods or any recommended diets you would like to follow.

Now, you have learned almost all the basics about rheumatoid arthritis diet, food preparation, and meal plans by reading this book. If you would like to know about other diets such as autoimmune paleo, low residue diets or fructose free diets, you can read the following books in the amazon kindle/paperback store written by the same author of this book:

The Autoimmune Paleo Cookbook and Action Plan: A Simple Guide to Paleo Autoimmune Protocol Diet to Reverse Autoimmune Disease and Heal Your Body, by Monet Manbacci, P.h.D., Available in Amazon Kindle and Paperback formats, 2020.

Low Residue Diet Cookbook: A Comprehensive Diet Guide and Cookbook with Over 130 Low Fiber Dairy Free Gluten Free Recipes for People with Crohn's Disease, Ulcerative Colitis and Diverticulitis, by Monet Manbacci, P.h.D., Available in Amazon Kindle and Paperback formats, 2020.

The Fructose Free Cookbook: A Comprehensive Diet Guide and Cookbook with Over 120 Delicious Recipes For People With Fructose Intolerance or Malabsorption, by Monet Manbacci, P.h.D., Available in Amazon Kindle & Paperback Formats, 2020.

The author of this book would like to thank you for reading this book and hope the book was helpful to you.

If you found this book useful or learned something from it, It would be much appreciated if you write a short review on the Amazon website.

The success of such books highly depends on your honest reviews. Your reviews can help the author improve the quality of this book in the next revisions. It can help other people to make informed decisions about reading this book as well.

If you have any feedback, comments or questions, feel free to email Monet Manbacci: monetmanbacci@gmail.com

Thanks again for your support!

Monet Manbacci, Ph.D., is the author of *"Ulcerative Colitis Comprehensive Diet Guide and Cookbook"*, *"The Comprehensive Guide to Crohn's Disease"*, and *"Ulcerative Colitis Journal"* Books. He is an IBD patient who has a Doctor of Philosophy (Ph.D.) degree in Applied Sciences and has been involved in academic and scientific research for more than 14 years.

OTHER BOOKS BY HEALTHVIEW PUBLISHERS:

Crohn's Disease Comprehensive Diet Guide and Cookbook, by Monet Manbacci, P.h.D., Available in Amazon Kindle & Paperback Formats, 2019.

The Comprehensive Guide to Crohn's Disease, All You Need to Know About Crohn's Disease, from Diagnosis to Management & Treatment, by Monet Manbacci, P.h.D., Available in Amazon Kindle & Paperback Formats, 2019.

Ulcerative Colitis Comprehensive Diet Guide and Cookbook, by Monet Manbacci, P.h.D., Available in Amazon Kindle & Paperback Formats, 2020.

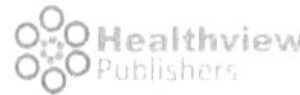